The Middle Age Doesn't Suck Guide To

Getting Fit and Staying Fit In Your 40s, 50s and Beyond

The Middle Age
Doesn't Suck Guide To

Getting Fit and
Staying Fit In Your
40s, 50s and Beyond

Jim Laabs

First American
Publishing

International Standard Book Number (ISBN-13) 978-0-976759-91-1

Printed in the United States of America

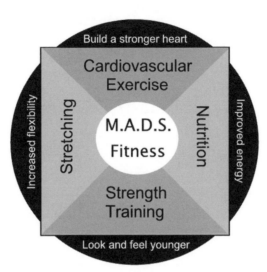

TABLE OF CONTENTS

Introduction

I'm sure you've heard this, because I've heard it more times than I can count – someone gives a middle-aged person a compliment that ends with the phrase, "for your age." As in, "You're in good shape – for your age." Or your doctor says, "This (insert condition here) is common for people your age."

It seems to me that once a person hits their late 40s, whatever physical decline a person experiences is often accepted as the natural course of aging. What's most troubling is that this acceptance applies not only to what others think, but that we even have a tendency to accept our own physical decline without a second thought. That's not right!

What's with the title "Middle Age Doesn't Suck"?

The MADS (Middle Age Doesn't Suck) books are dedicated to helping people in their 40s, 50s and 60s maximize this time of their life. Too often I see people hit middle age and start to settle for less, especially when it comes to health and fitness. I came up with the title, "Middle Age Doesn't Suck!" for shock value – I wanted to drive home the point that everyone can have a successful, fulfilling middle age.

A few words about my favorite subject: me

I got deeply involved in fitness about 10 years ago, when I was in my mid-40s. Physically, I was a wreck – I was 50 pounds overweight and looked a decade older than I was. Although I was athletic in my youth, walking to the garage to get in my car was my main exercise of the day.

Something – I don't recall what – inspired me to get into better shape and I started to gather every bit of information I could find about exercise and nutrition. By piecing together the stuff that worked and discarding the ideas that failed, I stumbled onto an exercise and nutrition program that works really great for people in their 40s through early 60s.

My results were outstanding – I lost weight and transformed my body within weeks. People who hadn't seen me for a couple of months were shocked. I still remember bumping into a fellow who was my long-time insurance agent. We had chatted for a few minutes when he asked if I was Jim's brother. He was quite embarrassed when he realized his mistake, but my appearance had really changed that much.

So, there I was – I had lost weight and gotten into fantastic shape. So why not do what everyone else does and write a book?

Just what the world needs: Another fitness book

The world doesn't need one more fitness book like all the others. There are already too many books about dieting and fitness that take themselves way too seriously. We have become a nation of joyless dieters and exercisers on a never-ending fitness treadmill that gets us nowhere. We grimly eat "light" foods that have the fun sucked out of them right along with the fat and calories – so we lose the enjoyment of eating but still don't succeed in losing weight.

I firmly believe that you can enjoy life while you're getting in shape. So I tried to make this book entertaining and easy to read. Hopefully you'll even have a few laughs as you read it. There's an old saying that goes, "The journey is more important than the destination." My wish for you is that you to succeed in whatever your fitness goals are – and that you have some fun while you're doing it.

In this book, I'll try to keep things simple. Too many fitness programs try to overwhelm people with science and details to the point where they are impossible to follow. The easiest plan to follow is one that you can understand and remember.

Don't expect much formality from these pages you are about to read. Once in awhile, I'll throw a fact or figure in to make a point but don't expect to find any footnotes. (Be honest: how often do you read footnotes, if ever? Footnotes are for suckers.) I hasten to add that you should not take my word as the gospel truth. I'm convinced that MADS fitness is a well designed plan that will produce great results for you, but I'll be the first to admit that I don't know all the answers. In fact, I'm pretty sure I don't even know all of the questions.

I joke around about being a "self-proclaimed fitness expert" but what it boils down to is that I'm a regular person, just like you, who doesn't have a full-time personal trainer or my own TV show. I got in shape the same way you do (or will), while balancing the pressures and responsibilities of day-to-day life. I started this program when I was in my mid-40s; so *I've been in the same place as you and I did it.* I've figured out a way to get in shape based on sound principles that works for people our age and think it's worthy of sharing what I've learned with you.

As you read the book, you'll find that I take some artistic license and use slang often. If you're prone to take offense you may be offended by my language. My apologies in advance; however, I suspect that I'm even worse in person. As long as I'm fessing up, I should also admit that I am a male, which is a blessing because I would be a very unattractive female. As I reviewed the manuscript for this book, I worried that I used too much of a male "voice" in my writing, which may lead female readers to mistakenly believe MADS is aimed at males. In fact, the MADS program works fantastically well for women, so please don't let my male-ness put you off.

But wait – there's more!

This book covers a lot of ground and gives you a complete program to follow. But like the infomercials say, "but wait – there's more!" Visit www.MADSfitness.com. You'll find recipes, advanced workout programs, different stretching routines, links and other neat stuff. As a reader who plunked down good money for this book, you'll have access to a whole bunch of premium content that non-readers will be locked out of, miserable pudknockers that they are.

Last but certainly not least: get started. Follow the MADS program as best you can. If you can't stick with it 100%, try for 90%. If you can't hit 90%, then shoot for 80%. Make changes in your diet and exercise, small or large – just keep getting better. Best wishes to you in reaching your fitness goals!

Jim Laabs

December, 2007

Chapter One

How you can feel and look younger with MADS fitness

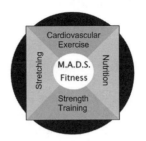

Since you didn't read the Introduction (who does?) I'll tell the story again how I stumbled across the fitness program described in this book after some trial and error (a lot of error). Before I discovered the MADS (Middle Age Doesn't Suck) system, I was a living example of unsuccessful dieting.

How about this for dieting success? Between the ages of 30 and 45, I lost over 100 pounds! The bad news is that they were the same pounds over and over again. Sometimes I'd lose 10 pounds; other times as much as 30 or 40 pounds. But I always put the weight back on again (plus a little extra) within months. That's one of the biggest problems with almost every weight loss program – at some point the diet stops and old habits kick back in. Unless there is a change in metabolism and eating habits, every weight loss program is doomed to fail sooner or later.

But MADS is different! For me, it has brought results. I lost 55 pounds, going from 247 to 192, and I can pretty much eat what I want (within limits, and I have been known to stretch the limits) and I'm for the most part able to maintain my weight in a manageable range.

Overcoming health problems of middle age

When I was in my pre-MADS days, I had more than my share of health complaints that I blamed on getting older. I had a "trick ankle" that tended to twist and sprain if I stepped on the slightest uneven surface like the edge of a sidewalk. I had a half-dozen painful ankle sprains every year because of it. Guess how many ankle sprains I have had since I took up the MADS program? Not a single one.

Be careful about reading health books.

You may die of a misprint.   Mark Twain

Another health complaint during my mid-40s was my lower back. I tried chiropractic treatments, muscle relaxing pills and everything else. What finally got rid of my back pain for good was getting on the MADS program.

If you're in your 40s, 50s or 60s there's a good chance that you have various nagging aches and pains in your feet, knees, legs and who knows where else. Like many people, you've probably blamed those aches and pains on the natural course of aging. But if you give the MADS system a chance you'll find that you can set back your body's clock. You'll be surprised at how many of those aches and pains will go away once the results of the MADS program take hold.

A chair and the MADS program: how are they alike?

To understand the MADS program, let's compare it to a chair. Sturdy chairs have four legs. If you take one leg away, you can probably still sit in the chair, but it will be pretty tippy. Take away another leg from the chair and you'll struggle to

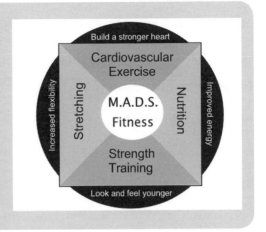

This diagram is a pesky way to keep reminding you how the four parts of the MADS program fit together and that strength training, cardio exercise, nutrition and stretching will all work together to help you get fit and healthy.

keep your balance. Try sitting on a one-legged chair and you'll be on the floor in no time at all.

The MADS system also has four "legs," and each leg is equally important. Follow all four parts of the MADS program and you'll be on the way to a healthy, fit lifestyle. Ignore one or more of the parts, and in the long run your fitness situation will be shaky at best. Here are the four parts of the MADS fitness system:

(1) Strength training: Builds muscle and avoids the muscle and bone mass loss that occurs over time. Strength training improves your "balance" muscles to help prevent falls and lessen your chances of injury. Strength training also gives you stamina and more energy so you'll feel better throughout the day.

(2) Cardiovascular exercise: This type of exercise strengthens your heart, lungs and circulatory system. Studies have shown that people who participate in even mild cardiovascular exercise on a regular basis are much less likely to have serious heart and circulatory problems. Cardio exercise also burns calories to help you lose or maintain your weight (depending on how many of those burned calories you replace with food!).

(3) Proper nutrition and eating habits: If you need to lose weight, you can't do it by exercise alone; eating right is also necessary. MADS will steer you to higher quality foods that will help you lose weight and help you to avoid foods that harm your health.

(4) Stretching: Frequent stretching helps relieve stiffness, improves flexibility and reduces a lot of common aches and pains.

I realize that facing a four-part fitness regimen looks intimidating. Part of your trepidation (if I may use a word that I'm not sure I even know the meaning of) is because you've been fed a line of continual B.S. from the various makers of diet pills, weight loss programs and infomercial exercise gizmos. You've been told thousands of times that getting into shape requires no work, no sweat and no time; all you need to do is get out your charge card.

I'm here to set things straight and give you the honest truth. In the long run, the only way to be at the weight you want, improve your overall health and live a longer, more active life is by following the principles laid out in this book.

When you confront a problem you

begin to solve it. Rudy Giuliani

If you're still reading and not looking for your receipt so you can return this book to your bookstore, I am glad to say that I just gave you the bad news. The good news is that we're going to get into shape and we'll even have some fun doing it. And don't worry – once you're in the swing of it, the program will seem pretty easy. And the effort will pay off in making you feel and look years younger.

How much commitment is required?

You might be saying to yourself, "I have a job and a life; how will I have time for all of this?" I'm not going to lie to you – MADS takes a few hours of exercise each week and a bit of planning about what kind of food you're going to be cramming into your yap on any particular day.

I might as well exercise; I'm already

in a bad mood anyway! Anonymous

However, I can tell you from my experience that my job or personal life haven't suffered one bit from exercising on a regular basis. I've had jobs where I've routinely worked 60 or more hours a week and still found time to exercise for five or six hours a week. The secret is to make it part of your routine.

The first three parts of the MADS system (strength, cardio and stretching) require a total of about four or five hours per week. You can certainly spend more time if you wish, but four to five hours will get the job done. Later in the book, I'll lay out a bunch of possible schedules for working out, and I'm willing to bet that one of those schedules will fit into your lifestyle.

The fourth part of MADS, the nutrition program, is easy to follow and doesn't involve any bizarre foods. You'll probably find many of the MADS-recommended foods in your fridge or pantry right now (along with some foods that you may have to get rid of – sorry about that).

Setting your fitness goals

When you embark on this (or any) fitness program, it's important for you to think about this question: what results are you looking for in order to feel like your efforts were successful?

> *Don't let anyone say you*
>
> *can't do it.* John Ilhan

I won't be so presumptuous as to set your goals for you but here are some ideas on how to set goals:

- Some goals can be specific while others can be general. For example, you may set a goal of losing 20 pounds in the next two months – that's a specific goal. A general goal may be to improve your appearance and look younger.

- When it comes to weight loss goals, sometimes it's better to avoid poundage loss as a goal and instead focus your goals on the benefits of losing weight. For instance, you may set a goal of fitting into a size 8 dress or cutting your waist size by four inches.

- It's fun to set "lifestyle and activity goals," where you aim to improve your lifestyle or be able to carry out an activity that you never would consider tackling in your current fitness state. I chose SCUBA diving as an activity goal and I was able to be active in diving after I got into shape.

• Always be realistic in setting goals…unfortunately, there isn't any program, including MADS, that will take you back to your teens again.

• Your goals don't have to be extreme; a lifestyle goal may be as simple as not feeling completely wiped out after an afternoon of shopping. Ask yourself: what are some things you would like to do if you were in better shape?

• The best approach is to have a couple goals aimed at things that you can measure, like inches off your waist or pounds lost, but be sure to have at least a couple of lifestyle and activity goals as well. It's the lifestyle goals that will give you an emotional stake in your fitness program.

OK – hopefully you're ready to go and have written down some goals. Enough of the preliminaries…let's get this party started and get healthy!

> *The miracle isn't that I finished. The miracle is*
> *that I had the courage to start.* John Bingham

Chapter Two

Strength training: Why bother?

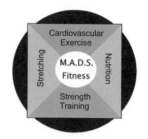

Big strong man

Big strong man

Picks up stuff

Just 'cause he can

- from the TV show "Wings"

In this section, we'll lay out basics of the Middle Age Doesn't Suck (MADS) system for strength training. If you've done strength training previously (or if you're doing it now) try to fight the urge to skip over any of this section. The strength training techniques that we will use are specifically geared for middle-agers and you just might find we do things a little differently than other strength training programs.

The first question you might ask is, "This looks like a lot of work. Why should I go through the time and trouble to do strength training?" If you're looking to turn back the clock (and aren't we all?) one of the very best things you can do is strength training.

Keep more muscle, keep more strength

The saying, "use it or lose it," is especially true when it comes to losing muscle as you age. People start losing muscle mass around age 40, and that loss speeds up as time passes. A proven way to put the brakes on muscle loss, according to several medical studies (none of which I feel like listing here), is to adopt a regular program of strength training.

What's wrong with muscle loss? Plenty! Less muscle means you tire more easily and are more susceptible to injury. Strength training will give you the strength you need so can stand longer without getting tired, walk further and maintain more energy throughout the day.

If you wait until all the lights are green

before you leave home, you'll never

get started on your trip. Zig Ziglar

Your body has dozens of unappreciated muscles that help your limbs react quickly when your brain tells them to. Getting these muscles into shape will increase how effectively these little muscles react, giving you better balance and faster reflexes.

Stronger bones

Like muscle, bones tend to lose their mass as we get older. The bones of a 70-year-old weigh considerably less than they did when that person was a young adult. That makes older bones more brittle and more susceptible to breaking.

The good news is that strength training not only slows muscle loss, it slows bone loss as well. Strength training is like a wake-up call, telling your body to keep those bones strong because there's still hard work to be done. Besides working out, it's important to include calcium in your diet since that's the building material your body needs to answer strength training's wake-up call.

Easier weight control

One of the pleasant surprises of the MADS system is the jump-start that strength training gives your body's metabolism. When it comes to burning energy, muscle is like a powerful blast furnace while fat is like a little tiny match. After you replace some of your fat with muscle, you'll be surprised at how you can eat more and not put on weight. (Assuming you eat the right kinds of foods – not even the MADS program is a free pass to eating unlimited donuts!)

Lose lots of inches, not just pounds

I'm a dieting expert (having done it so many times), and let me tell you, until you try the MADS program, you haven't seen the awesome loss of size that can be accomplished with the right combination of diet and truly effective exercise.

When you dance, your purpose is not to

get to a certain place on the floor. It's to enjoy

each step along the way. Wayne Dyer

MADS makes you lose more inches largely because of strength training. Why? Pound for pound, muscle takes up a lot less space than fat, and toned-up muscles are more compact than out-of-condition muscles. The combined effect of fat loss, muscle toning and muscle gain can be extraordinary. When I first discovered MADS I went from a 40-inch waistline to a 33-inch waistline in just ten weeks.

Bulk versus strength

I'll bet many of you are concerned that strength training will result in huge, Incredible Hulk-like muscles. You worry that you'll fall into addiction to muscle-building food additives, spiraling into use of illegal anabolic steroids and end up named in a tell-all book by some former baseball player and steroid junkie. Trust me, you won't grow huge muscles overnight if you follow the MADS methods.

I really don't think I need buns of steel. I'd be

happy with buns of cinnamon. Ellen DeGeneres

All kidding aside, here are the facts. Testosterone (that's a hormone) is a necessary ingredient for building big muscles. Young men have it practically coming out of their ears and they tend to build muscle quickly from strength training. Young women produce testosterone, but in smaller amounts, so weight training usually doesn't cause much muscle growth in females.

Starting in their 40s, men start to produce less testosterone than they did when they were younger, and women produce very little of the hormone. That's why people start to lose muscle in middle age, and the loss gets progressively worse. So strength training is important because you can head off the loss of muscle and even add a bit extra.

The Body Area Workout that we use in MADS is designed to add strength without adding extra bulk. Generally, the way to build big muscles is to do a low number of reps with heavier weights. Body builder types may do three sets of a very small number of reps with really heavy weights. The way to build strength and stamina is to use low-to-moderate weights and moderate-to-high reps (like three sets of 10 to 12 reps each), which is what we generally do in MADS.

More core strength means a better you

A big reason why we middle-agers get tired and have aches and pains is dwindling "core strength." Most people look at strength as having huge, sinewy (I never imagined I'd use the word "sinewy" in a normal sentence) arms and legs. But there are all kinds of important muscles between your shoulders and hips that help you move around throughout the day. The MADS program works on strengthening those muscles. After you develop more core strength with MADS you'll find that you have better balance, more stamina, improved coordination, and generally feel more physically centered.

A person too busy to take care of their

health is like a mechanic too busy

to take care of his tools. Spanish proverb

I hope you're convinced that there are plenty of fantastic reasons to try out strength training, because those are all the reasons I know. Let's find out how to get started.

Chapter Three:

The Body Area Workout

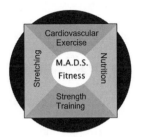

Before we begin, let me set out some principles that I'll try to stick to. First, we're going to keep it simple. Many people in the fitness biz tend to make this stuff more mysterious and complicated than it really is. As a result, I see many people our age carrying notes around with them while they work out so that they can remember what to do next. Have these folks already started to lose their power of memory? No, I think it's that they were given too much to think about.

Another thing I'll try to do is talk about why you do a certain exercise instead of just giving you a list of exercises, without you even knowing why you're doing them. If you see the big picture, you'll enjoy it more be more motivated because you'll better understand why you're spending all this time pushing and pulling weights.

Finally, let's make this fun. Strength training doesn't have to be a chore, and I want to get you excited about it.

All set? Then let's go!

Know your body parts

You probably think you're already intimately familiar with your body parts, at least the important ones. But for our purposes, we are going to look at your body parts as they pertain to strength training. We'll simplify how we talk about muscle groups. There are a bunch of scientific names for muscles and we could spend several pages talking about them, but we're just going to call them by the main name, like biceps, and leave it at that.

Assuming that your head is properly attached to your body at this moment, look down and you'll hopefully find your legs. We're concerned about three groups of muscles in the legs. Starting from the bottom, your calf muscles are below your knees and in back of your legs. For our purposes, they extend around to the front of your legs and include your shins. Staying behind your knee but moving up, the muscle group between your rear end and your knees are your hamstrings, which I call "hammies." Around the front are your thighs, which are sometimes called your "quads," short for quadriceps.

These are not the only muscles in the vicinity of your legs that will end up getting a workout, because muscles in the hips, feet, butt and so forth are going to come along for the ride and get in shape whether they like it or not.

Moving north of your waist, the fancy word for the area between your waist and shoulders is the "core," so I will be a fancy man and call it that. Located in the back core is (as you probably guessed) your back. In front you have your chest muscles, and between your chest and down into your waist area are your abdominal muscles, which in fitness lingo are called "abs."

Finally, look to your left and right and you'll find your arms. If you looked and did not see them, please look again and locate two of them before reading further. We're not going to worry about the part of the arm below the elbow, because frankly, what has it done for us lately? Actually, we have in the forearms, wrists, and hands some more muscles that we won't work directly, but they will end up getting worked indirectly.

Don't quack like a duck...soar like an eagle. Ken Blanchard

We *will* worry about what's above the elbows, where we have two important muscle groups. Pretend for a moment that you're Governor Ah-nold of Cal-ee-for-nee-uh and flex for all it's worth. The part that's supposed to be bulging hugely upward is your biceps. The back side of your upper

In case you weren't keeping count, we've taken the many muscles in your body and simplified them down to just nine. Here they are:

Legs:

Calves

Hamstrings

Quads (thighs)

Core area:

Back

Chest

Abs

Shoulders and arms:

Shoulders

Biceps

Triceps

arm (opposite from the biceps) is the triceps group of muscles. Located between your arms and your head are your shoulders, which are surrounded all around by a group of muscles that fitness folks call deltoids or "delts" for short.

Which parts do we work and when?

Here is a big way in which MADS differs with conventional wisdom, a nice way of saying "what other self-proclaimed fitness experts will tell you." In MADS we try to involve every body part in each workout. That's worth repeating, so go ahead and repeat it – in the meantime I'll start writing the next sentence.

The whole MADS strength training philosophy is based on understanding the different body areas, and then using this knowledge to set up your own workout schedule that best fits your time limitations and fitness goals.

I think you get more health benefit and personal satisfaction by working all nine muscle groups every time you work out.

A complete workout is ideal, but if you are pressed for time, we'll explain how to split your workouts between upper body and lower body (arms, shoulders and chest one time, back, legs and abs the next; better yet, do your abs in both work-outs). In a nearly perfect world, you would work every group at least twice a week; in a *really* perfect world, it would be three times per muscle group per week.

Reps and sets

The words "reps" (short for repetitions) and "sets" (a short word all on its own) are important strength training terms. A rep is going through one complete motion of moving a weight forward and back (or back and forward depending on the exercise). We repeat this motion a number of times, and that collection of reps is called a set. So if someone tells you they did "3 sets of 10 reps," they performed the complete motion for that exercise 10 times, rested a minute, did it 10 more times, rested, then finished with 10 final reps. The total number of reps in this example is 30, with one-minute rest periods sandwiched in between sets of 10.

For each exercise we do, we'll generally shoot for three sets ranging from 8 to 15 reps each, depending on the type of workout we're doing.

Rest between sets

How long should you rest between sets? A good guideline is about one minute. Less than a minute might not leave you with enough gas to finish all your sets, and if you go any longer than that, you're mistaking the weight bench for a park bench. (Just kidding; it's no crime to go beyond a minute once in awhile but try to keep the rest period no longer than 1-1/2 minutes at the very most.)

You'll eventually develop a feel for the timing and your body will tell you when you should start the next set. Some people wear a watch to keep tight control of their rest times, but that's too much precision for me, so I just guesstimate. If you don't time your rests, try not to get caught up in conversation or daydreaming that results in several minutes going by between sets.

Rest between workouts

While you're puffing and straining during your workout, your muscles are taking quite a beating. In fact, they are actually developing little tiny tears (some-times called micro-tears) that need time to heal. As they heal, the muscle cells grow in reaction to the stress you put on them and you get bigger and/or stronger muscles. Rest between workouts is important because muscles heal on your rest days. That's why it's important to never work the same muscle group twice without a minimum of two nights sleep in between.

Try to hit all muscle groups in every workout, but...

My favorite schedule is "all or nothing." I like to do all my strength training in one workout, take the next day off (maybe do some walking and some abdominal exercises), then do a complete strength workout again the following day. This "all or nothing" approach requires about a solid hour of gym time, and if you do cardio at the same time (which I like to do), you need to set aside about 1-1/2 hours of gym time. I allow two hours door-to-door, including getting gussied up after my workout and drive time to and from.

I better explain the "all or nothing" term I used, because I may have just provided some of you with a nice excuse to choose "nothing." I have tried it all ways, and have found that an every-other-day-entire-workout-all-at-one-time approach is more effective at boosting metabolism than other schedules.

I have used a "split" schedule, breaking the strength training portion in half and working out almost every day, and for me it doesn't work nearly as well. I experience better results in terms of muscle development, I feel lots better and my metabolism seems considerably faster when I do a full workout every other day. It may not seem like it on first glance, but the every-other-day approach saves time as well, especially if you work out at a gym.

❗ MADS Tip!

Here's an example of the time required for a full body versus split workout, assuming 15 minutes before and after each workout to get to and from:

Full body workout...

Work out 3 to 4 times per week; each workout consists of full body strength training plus 25-30 minutes cardio exercise (Monday-Wednesday-Friday-Sunday, etc.)

Average door-to-door time spent per workout = 2 hours

Time investment with travel = 6 to 8 hours per week

Split workouts in half...

Work out 6 days per week with half-workouts - each workout consists of half body strength training plus 20 minutes cardio exercise

Average door-to-door time spent per workout = 1-1/2 hours

Time investment with travel = 9 hours per week

But I'm a realist if nothing else. I understand that real life may demand that you split your workout. So, set a workout schedule that works for you; one that you will stick with on a regular basis. That's the most important thing. You are better off splitting your workout than not doing it at all.

Say hello to your new friend, muscle soreness

I hate to break some bad news to you, but you'll probably get sore muscles from strength training, at least in the early going. The stress of strength training causes those tiny tears we talked about to occur in the muscle fibers, which in turn causes inflammation and releases stuff called "fatigue acids" during the healing process. These acids are what cause muscle soreness.

If you are sore, be sure to take a full day off before working those muscles again – but don't skip your next scheduled workout! You might walk into your next workout still sore from two days before, but after you finish that workout, your soreness often will feel much better. It's kind of like "the hair of the dog" for a hangover – the movement of the muscles forces the fatigue acids out of the muscle tissue and into the bloodstream, where they are dissolved.

How long your muscle soreness lasts depends on your body and how hard you are pushing things. If you frequently increase the amount of weight you are using, you may have to accept being a little sore as part of your daily life. (Being extremely sore or having soreness in your joints as opposed to muscles is not a good thing anytime, and probably indicates that you have overdone it).

In MADS we take very definite steps to minimize soreness in the early going, but unfortunately, it can't be eliminated.

I've got to tell a story that I've kept to myself for quite a while. When my youngest daughter was in college, I had a trick I used a couple of times. My daughter would meet boys at school or while we were on vacation, and in a couple of instances these young men decided to travel great distances to visit her for a few days in the city where we lived. I would make it a point to schedule a workout the first day that her male friend arrived, and offer to take him with me to the gym as my guest.

My workout was aggressive and used relatively heavy weights. I discouraged these eager young men from trying to keep up with me, but their egos usually won out and they would (predictably) try to follow my routine. (It can't be that hard for a 20-year-old to keep up with a bald middle-aged guy, right?) Well, just as predictable as their egos was the result, which was intense – and I mean intense – muscle soreness. Hopefully, romance was the last thing on these guys' minds for the next day or two.

Understanding progressive resistance

MADS strength training is based on a principle called progressive resistance. The resistance (the amount of weight you lift) slowly increases (progresses) over weeks and months. A simple concept, but to really carry out progressive resistance requires a degree of self discipline. At our advanced age, self discipline is a quality we are supposed to have in abundance, so I guess we're in luck.

In MADS, we start with minimal weight, and slowly add small amounts of weight over a number of weeks and months. For example, for a particular exercise you might add 2-1/2 or 5 pounds every week or two if you feel your muscles have adapted to the old weight. Adding weight slowly helps prevent injuries, but still gives you the results you want from all that work you're doing.

I have to exercise early in the morning before my

brain figures out what I am doing. Unknown

To minimize muscle soreness and chance of injury with any new exercise movement, your first session should be with minimal weight, 10-20 pounds or less.

The second time that you perform an exercise you should increase the weight to a level that offers noticeable resistance, but does not make you strain whatsoever at the end of a set. This would be about 50% of the weight you think you'll end up lifting once you start going full steam.

On your third time with a particular exercise, bump up the weight by 5 pounds. Increase the weight by 5 pounds (or less) each session until the last rep of the last set (see why we learned those fitness terms?) is difficult to do. However, you should be able to complete that last rep without losing your good form and without excessive strain. If you add too much weight and you can't finish your planned reps in each set, take off a little weight the next time.

Every week or so, re-evaluate your progress and how much weight you should be using. Add a little weight if you think your sets are getting too easy.

The main reason we start with low weights is so that you become accustomed to the proper motion for that exercise before you add lots of weight, which minimizes the chance of extreme soreness and injury.

You'll find in the early going that you can add weight pretty often, as often as once a week. As the weeks and months pass by, you won't be able to add weight as frequently and eventually you'll go for months without adding weight. But always try to make progress.

Be careful on new machines

If you switch machines or go to a different gym, keep in mind that not all equipment is equal. You may be able to bench press 100 pounds on one machine, and on another bench press machine even 80 pounds will be impossible. Be careful and start with low weights whenever you use a new machine for the first time.

Which exercises come first?

There's a right order for exercises. All you need to remember is: (1) Work opposing body parts (muscles on your front and then those on the back) one after another, and (2) work large muscles before small muscles.

Let's look at opposing body parts first. Remember our muscle groups we came up with? The three major groups are: (1) legs, (2) arms, and (3) core. When we say you work opposing muscles, you are staying in the same major group, working a front muscle, then a back muscle. For example, if you work your hamstrings (the back of your legs), you would next want to work your quads (front of legs). Next, you would work your calves to finish your legs, and then you would move onto another muscle group.

If you're having trouble visualizing front and back, first attempt to twist your head completely backwards. If that doesn't work, refer to the following chart:

Opposing muscles: Front versus back

! MADS Tip!

Part	Front	Back
Legs	Thighs	Hamstrings
	Quadriceps	
Core	Chest	Upper back
	Abdominals	Lower back
Arms	Biceps	Triceps

Shoulders have fronts and backs too, but they aren't true opposing muscles so we'll throw those in and work them in the same group as the arms. Here's the general order we work our muscles:

1. Quads and hamstrings

2. Calves

3. Abdominal muscles

4. Chest and back muscles

5. Shoulders

6. Upper arms

7. Forearms

If you don't have this order stuff down yet, don't worry about it. We'll set up some workouts later that will give you a clear idea of the correct order.

Technique is more important than lots of weight

If you decide to work out at a gym, you'll notice this sooner rather than later: Some guy (usually it's only guys who are guilty of this) has a humongous amount of weight that he is working with. He's making sounds unlike anything heard in nature as he moves the weights so fast they are rattling. Since you are a newbie in the gym, you feel inferior and start to feel like you need to keep up and add more weight to what you are lifting.

This little story makes two points. First: Never worry about what the person next to you is doing. How much weight they lift or how fast they run on the treadmill doesn't mean a thing. Everyone has their own story and countless reasons why they are doing more (or less) than you.

Here's the second thing to remember: Always lift the amount of weight that you feel comfortable with, but enough to offer a challenge. Resist the temptation to go for more weight than you are ready for. Staying within your capabilities is the best way to avoid injuries.

Never eat more than

you can lift. Miss Piggy

One of our main goals in MADS is to keep you exercising on a regular basis. Getting hurt will put you out of commission for a long time. Practicing good form with the right amount of weight minimizes the chance you'll end up with some complaint that keeps you away from exercising for weeks or months.

I'm going to summarize what was said earlier because it is vitally important: Start with very low resistance during the first session in which you do a new exercise so that you can get a feel for the proper motion. The next session, you can increase the weight to a higher level, but low enough so you can still finish all your sets without straining at all (50% of the weight you think you'll eventually be lifting). During the third session, increase the weight by 5 pounds and keep increasing the amount each workout until you find it challenging to finish the last rep or two of the final set. Then increase weights by small amounts as your sets get too easy. But always, always maintain proper technique. What is proper technique? It consists of three things: (1) form, (2) pace, and (3) breathing.

Form

Every exercise has a right way to do it and countless wrong ways. Performing an exercise the wrong way usually results in you not getting full benefit from the exercise, or worse yet, getting injured. Paying strict attention to proper form isn't just for beginners. Every single time I go to the gym I see at least one example of absolutely horrendous form, and too often it is a middle-aged person.

It has been my observation that most

people get ahead during the time that

others waste time. Henry Ford

A good way to check your form is if your workout area has mirrors. After you're done posing and flexing, look at your form as you exercise. Another way to check your form is whether you feel the effects of the exercise in the targeted muscles. If you've just finished doing leg curls and your abs are tired but your quads are not, you are probably doing something wrong.

In the Appendix you'll find suggested strength training exercises, including tips for each exercise to help you use proper form.

Pace

One of the most common ways to "cheat" and fool yourself is to go through the lifting motion faster than you should. The momentum you create helps you lift more weight than you otherwise could so you can convince yourself that you're stronger than you really are.

What's a good pace? Shoot for 1-1/2 to 2 seconds up (on the hard part of the exercise, often referred to as the "positive") and about 2 seconds down (the easier part of the exercise, often called the "negative"). Use the old "one-one-thousand-two-one-thousand" count to get a feel for the pace. Or better yet, you can repeat the phrase, "Jim is a fitness god, Jim is a fitness god." Be sure to check your pace every once in a while to make sure you haven't slipped into any bad habits.

You should include a very brief pause (a fraction of a second) in your lifting motion at the bottom of the motion. When you let the weight back down, you should pause briefly at the bottom before pushing it up again. This dispels the momentum and makes sure you have to use all that new-found muscle of yours to get that weight back up again.

Breathing

Are you starting to think "Holy cow, you said you were going to keep this simple!"? Remember, we're laying out the whole shootin' match here. We'll summarize all of this stuff pretty soon and boil it down to a few basics that even I have been able to remember, so you should be able to remember it as well.

Anyway, let's talk about breathing. There are two main points to remember about breathing: (1) Never hold your breath, in other words always breath naturally, and (2) Exhale as you are doing the lifting (positive) part of the motion, and inhale on the easier (negative) part of the motion.

The way to get started is to quit

talking and begin doing. Walt Disney

If you hold your breath, the air in your lungs coupled with the strain of lifting can cause various injuries. And who is silly enough to do this? Just about everyone at one time or another, including me. In my case, I ended up with a slightly torn esophagus, which gave me some pretty painful heartburn for a few days, so I learned to always think about my breathing when lifting.

The old timers like Charles Atlas used to say, "Blow the weight up," to remember to exhale at the right time. The proper phrase should actually be something like "exhale in a controlled fashion the weight up," but that doesn't sound nearly as snappy. The point is you really should not try to blow, simply exhale as you normally would during the "hard" part of the motion.

Warming up

If the first part of your workout is strength training, you will need to warm up a bit before hitting the heavy weights. Warming up gets the blood moving through your muscles, which will make them less susceptible to pulls, tears and strains, none of which you want to happen. There are several options for warming up:

(1) Do a quick set of 10 reps of your first few strength exercises with very little weight. If your first exercise is the leg curl, you might do a set of 10 reps with 10 or 20 pounds, and then perform your three regularly scheduled sets with normal weight. You don't need to do this for every exercise, just the first three or four.

(2) Walk briskly for about five minutes, being sure to move your arms a little more than you would in normal walking.

(3) Do five minutes on a cardio machine at a moderate pace.

Injuries and illness

Our philosophy is to try like heck to avoid getting injured – but muscle strains, tendonitis, smooshed fingers and various other injuries occasionally happen.

Our rules for avoiding injury are simple:

1. Use an amount of weight that you are comfortable with

2. Pay attention to your form, pace and breathing at all times

3. If you feel pain, especially in a joint, skip that exercise!

 MADS Tip!

You should avoid certain exercises to minimize chances of injury. The biggest offenders are the clean and jerk, dead lift, snatch and traditional squats. We won't even talk about the first three (although I suspect many people think of me as a jerk and I hope I'm clean) and we'll be extremely careful doing squats.

I'm not into working out. My philosophy:

No pain, no pain. Carol Leifer

Unfortunately, injuries do happen. For middle-agers, the most common is joint problems. An effective treatment for tendonitis, sore knees, hips and pulled muscles is to apply ice for about 10 minutes at a time once every 30 minutes. Use ice treatments for a few days after the injury or pain occurs, then try switching to heat.

Ice relieves the inflammation and helps speed the healing process during the early stages of recuperation; heat helps the healing process once inflammation is in check. If heat doesn't help or makes it feel worse, try returning to icing. Generally, tendonitis responds better to icing. Don't work out (or only work other body parts) until you can exercise the injured area with very minimal or no pain.

When should you skip a workout due to illness? If you have a fever you should not work out. If your doctor advises you to rest due to illness or injury, follow the advice. If you think you're coming down with something, think not only about yourself but others. Going to the gym when you are contagious is not a nice thing to do to your fellow gym rats. If you have a cold but have passed the first couple of days when you are contagious and feel all right, it's generally OK to work out.

But, always (whether you are sick or not) wipe down equipment with the disinfectant provided after you are finished using it.

Is there any end to this chapter?

Yes. Let's simplify all this and give you just 5 things to remember:

1. Always practice proper form, pace and breathing.

2. Use the amount of weight that challenges you to finish 3 sets of your chosen number of reps each.

3. Slowly increase the amount of weight you use by small increments as completing the sets becomes too easy.

4. If your schedule permits, work all body parts in each workout. If you can't do everything, split into 2 workouts to cover all parts. If that doesn't work, go to 3 workouts and work each muscle group twice a week.

5. Work opposing body parts in the same group together, and work large muscles before small muscles.

That's it – 5 "rules of the road" to a safe, workable strength training program that will give you outstanding results!

> *It's easy to have faith in yourself and*
> *have discipline when you're a winner,*
> *when you're number one. What you've*
> *got to have is faith and discipline when*
> *you're not yet a winner.* Vince Lombardi

Chapter Four:

To gym or not to gym? That is the question

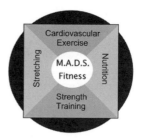

O ne of the most frequent questions I hear is, "Should I get a gym member-ship or buy equipment to use at home?" I myself am a "gym guy" and, in my humble-but-self-proclaimed-expert opinion, working out at a gym is easier, safer, funner (note to my second grade English teacher: I do know that "funner" is not a real word), more economical and more likely to give you better results than working out at home.

But the decision of working out at home or in a gym is one you'll have to make for yourself, sport, so I'll do my best to lay out the pluses and minuses.

In terms of economics, a home gym costs $1,000 minimum and can easily end up at $3,000 or more. Assuming a good gym in your area has memberships for $40 to $60 a month, you could get about two years at a gym for the cost of the most economical home gym.

Working against health clubs is the cost and time of driving to and from the gym. Unless it's a very convenient location for you, the back-and-forth can add up to lots of mileage and hours over the months and years.

MADS Tip! Work out at home or gym?	
Home	**Gym**
No travel time or gas cost	Mileage and driving time
Less variety of equipment	More choice of equipment
No professional trainer	Trainer usually on site
Equipment repairs your worry	Someone else maintains it
Solitary, no social atmosphere	Other people are around
Pick your own music and TV	The gym's TV and music
Upfront equipment cost	Monthly payments
Equipment is always available	May have to wait for equipment

I'm not really an accountant but I play one in this book

Excuse me a moment, I'm putting my accountant pants on. OK, I'm ready to talk like an accountant... Let's use your favorite author (that would be me) as an example. I belonged to a gym that was located a little over six miles out of my way on my way home from work. I went there an average of three times a week. I belonged to that gym for over four years so that's over 600 round trips of 12 miles each, which is 7,200 miles. At 30 cents a mile for gas and wear-and-tear, it cost me $2,160 to drive to and from the gym. That made my *true cost* of belonging to that gym equal to the $40 monthly fee plus over $45 per month in travel costs, for a total of $85 per month.

The decision is more than just dollars

Whew, my brain is tired and I think I smell smoke. I'm taking off my accounting pants now, because obviously there's much more to this decision than just dollars. One of the key things to think about is: Will you feel comfortable in a gym? Some people feel right at home in a health club and some don't. But, if you're worried about not looking trim and fit amongst all of the trim and fit members, don't be concerned. Plenty of un-trim and un-fit people inhabit gyms.

The best way to evaluate a gym is to visit at the time of day that you would normally work out. Check out the crowds, how available equipment is and the general condition of the place. In terms of condition, look for tell-tale signs like torn cushions on equipment, "out of order" signs on equipment, few available machines and dust bunnies in corners. These are signs of poor maintenance or too many members for the equipment available.

Different gyms tend to have different personalities. You may find one gym is where all the body builders work out while another one has a larger base of women, maybe because they offer more aerobics classes. That brings up a good point – if you are interested in aerobics or other classes, make sure your gym offers them when you are able to attend. Ask for a schedule of classes of all kinds.

The social aspect of gyms is the proverbial two-edged sword. On one hand, it relieves the day-to-day rut you may find yourself in. And depending on your preferences, you may like to be around other people during your workout. On the

Gym Etiquette

I have seen some wacky behavior in gyms. Always one to see the glass as half-full, I will give my fellow mankind the benefit of the doubt and assume they are not acting like jackasses on purpose but out of ignorance of proper gym etiquette. In that spirit, I outline these suggestions to follow in order to avoid annoying your fellow man (I mean that in a gender non-specific way) while working out at a gym:

There is a custom in gyms called "working in." If someone asks you, "Can I work in?" they want to share the machine you are currently using. The polite response is to say, "Of course," with a pleasant smile. If you are starting your last set on that machine, it's OK to respond with something on the order of, "I just have one more set, and then it's all yours."

Don't camp out too long on one machine. Save conversations and long rests for when you are finished with a particular apparatus, and not between sets.

If you use a machine, bench or cardio machine and leave perspiration on it, wipe it off with either your own towel or one of the towels many gyms provide for that purpose. Many gyms provide a disinfectant spray – use it.

If you're using a bar or machine that uses weight plates, always remove the weight plates when you are finished and replace them on the storage rack provided.

It's OK to carry a small towel, a bottle of water and iPod-type device around the gym with you, but coats, clothes, car keys and other personal belongings should be stored in a locker. Not only do you keep the gym from looking like the floor of my closet, but you'll enjoy your workout more it you're not dragging stuff around.

Speaking of cell phones…multitasking is acceptable and sometimes necessary in today's world. But who wants to listen to a person a few feet away having a string of obviously unnecessary personal conversations that could easily be put off until later?

If your gym has individual TVs, keep the sound muted unless you are using headphones. People near you may not be watching the same program as you and your audio will be extremely annoying to them.

Shouting, loud groaning, and screaming are not proper behavior anywhere but in the bedroom, and certainly are not proper in a gym. A few old-timers still think it's cool to scream or shout to help them complete that last rep; don't follow their example.

other hand, there may be times when you are in a rush and want to get through your workout, or you have a problem at work that you want to ruminate about (note to readers in Brooksville, Florida – "ruminate" means "think") while you do your cardio. But, oops, here comes Mrs. Jones, and you know she's going to bend your ear for the entire time you're on the treadmill.

 MADS Tip!

What to look for in a gym

If you decide to join a gym, look for one that:

- Is conveniently located for you

- Is clean and has well-maintained equipment

- Has monthly rates and contract terms you can live with

- Is in synch with your personality and exercise goals

Also, I don't know how to put this delicately, so let me just say that there can be some real jackasses hanging out at gyms. There are people who don't wipe off the equipment so it's covered with their sweat when you sit down on it. (ick) And the guys who don't take their 45-pound weights off the machine when they are done. (I'm sure they think, "Why not leave hundreds of pounds of weights on this machine just in case the 98-pound woman who's going to use it next wants to lift that much weight?") And there are the three buddies that monopolize one piece of equipment for a half hour while they take turns using it, chatting for five minutes between sets while they lean on the machine.

I don't go to the gym. And the closest thing I have to

a nutritionist is the Carlsberg Beer Company. Colin Farrell

If you like being around other people, gyms can keep you interested in exercising. I personally find it motivating to work out at a gym because on any given day there are people at the gym who are a little further along the fitness road than me, but there are also some people that I am ahead of. That makes me feel good about how far I've come but reminds me that there is room for improvement.

One of the big advantages that a gym membership offers in the long run is variety. Gyms usually have a choice of two, three or more machines for doing a particular exercise, so you can approach your muscles from slightly different angles each workout. Also, the variety of different machines keeps you from getting bored.

Stick with the pros so you don't get conned

There is a breed of gyms that have multiplied like bunnies in recent years, but thank goodness seem to be declining in popularity. These gyms are often aimed at women but some are open to both sexes. They typically have no showers or dressing rooms, and most use a specifically defined circuit of equipment that you are supposed to follow.

Some of the equipment in these gyms doesn't even allow you to change the resistance, but you are told to move faster to increase the intensity of the exercise. I know a woman with no previous elbow problems who developed tendonitis after just a few weeks of using this type of equipment, and the symptoms disappeared soon after she stopped visiting that gym.

There is a reason these gyms sprang up so quickly: they can be opened by entrepreneurs for a fraction of the cost of a full service gym. The gym owner makes money and you're the one who pays the price. You'll be forced to use equipment that is designed to save the gym owner money rather than provide you with quality workout.

These gyms are usually staffed by minimum wage counselors with little or no fitness background. Contrast that to a full service gym where you generally receive two or three free sessions from a qualified personal trainer who will demonstrate how to use the equipment and help you set up a workout schedule.

Don't be too timid and squeamish about your actions.

All life is an experiment. Ralph Waldo Emerson

I need to differentiate the gyms I just described with another type of fitness center that is becoming popular. Personal trainers are not only flexing their biceps but are beginning to flex their business muscles and open their own training gyms. Often these are small gyms and some have limited facilities, but unlike the ones I mentioned earlier, these are legitimate gyms that offer the advantage of more accessibility to a personal trainer than you would have at a large, full-service health club. If you want to belong to a quality gym, but the hugeness of a big health club doesn't appeal to you, look into a smaller gym that is operated by certified personal trainers.

Opening a quality, full service gym requires an investment of hundreds of thousands of dollars for locker rooms and top notch equipment, not to mention high overhead for staff during the long hours a gym must be open. Gyms do go out of business, but you can usually count on a full service gym to be there for you year after year.

That concludes the lecture for today. I'd better step off my soapbox and catch my breath so we can talk about equipment.

Using weight machines properly

MADS Tip!

The weight machines sold for home use and found in gyms seem pretty self-explanatory, but there are plenty of ways to use machines incorrectly. Improper use may cause soreness or injury, or at the very least, shortchange you on the benefits you should get from using the machine. Here are some tips for using weight machines:

If the exercise movement involves bending your legs, arms or waist, figure out where the pivot point of the machine is and align that with the joint you are bending. On many machines the pivot point is denoted by a dot or other mark. Example: if you're doing arm curls, the joint you bend is your elbow. When you rest your arms on the machine's pad, the pivot point should be lined up with your elbows.

Most machines at the gym have a little instruction sign somewhere on them with a diagram showing the general motion for the exercise. If you buy a home exercise machine, it should come with a booklet demonstrating the various exercises possible.

A great way to learn to use an unfamiliar machine is to inconspicuously watch someone who looks like they know what they are doing. It's also OK to ask someone that you see using a machine how to adjust settings.

Always take time to adjust the seat height, seatback and any other settings to make sure that you are in proper position for the exercise.

If you join a health club, you may be offered a couple of sessions with a personal trainer. Use this free perk to have the trainer demonstrate and explain the machines that you would like to use.

A common way to unconsciously cheat on machines is to shorten the range of motion. Pay attention to where you start and stop your motion and make sure to carry through the full range of motion of the exercise.

Don't clank the weights down against the other weights every time you do a rep. Letting the weights hit each other is bad for the machine and it annoys your fellow man (or woman). It also demonstrates loudly that you're a novice.

Never, ever bounce. Your motion should always be smooth and controlled, and at a slow pace. Bouncing and jerky movements can cause injury.

Chapter Five

Choosing the right equipment for you

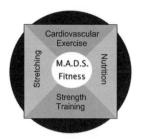

We're going to take a quick tour through the various options you have, whether at home or in a gym, for strength training equipment. Basically, the main choice in equipment is between free weights or machines.

"Free weights" are called that because they allow you unlimited freedom of movement. Free weights consist of either barbells or dumbbells. A barbell is a bar about four feet long with weights on both ends. Dumbbells are smaller, a foot or so long and they usually come in pairs, one for each hand. Both barbells and dumbbells have their place in the world of free weights but dumbbells seem more popular with the fitness crowd these days.

If free weights aren't your thing, then weight machines are for you. Weight machines come in a variety of shapes and sizes but they all use weights (or some other form of resistance) attached to cables. By and large, health clubs have machines that use a cable and pulley set-up to allow you to move actual stacks of weights. Home machines may use actual weights or another form of resistance.

Let's compare free weights to weight machines. If you are joining a gym, you will probably have access to both free weights and machines, but if you are planning to set up a home gym, you will most likely have to choose one or the other (or else plan to open up your wallet extra wide to buy both).

What does the self-proclaimed fitness god have to say?

I have been strength training for several years now, and machines still make up the vast majority of my routine. Once in awhile I use dumbbells during a workout and I hardly ever touch a barbell.

When I work out with free weights I'm conservative about how much weight I use for safety reasons. I'm not comfortable using a spotter, who is a person that stands by to catch the weight if you lose control of it. When people ask me to spot for them, I'd like to say, "Are you crazy? Don't you know how irresponsible I am?" but what comes out of my mouth is, "OK, sure..." Then I spend the next few minutes inches away from some sweaty guy (not surprisingly, attractive women never ask me to spot for them) listening to him grunt and strain, praying that he won't drop the weight and if he does drop it that I'll catch it and not have to live with the memory of his squashed face haunting me for the rest of my life.

Take care with free weights

If you're using free weights, be conservative in deciding how much weight to use. Dropping or losing control of free weights can lead to serious injury.

MADS Tip!

Free weights or weight machine?

Advantages and disadvantages of each

- Free weights exercise the small, "stability" muscles more than machines, because you have to balance the weights while you lift them.

- Machines limit you to a certain movement, while a pair of dumbbells can be used for dozens of different exercises.

- Free weights are considerably harder for beginners to use. I recommend that beginning strength trainers use machines for at least the first few months of training.

- There is greater risk of injury with free weights. You can drop free weights on various body parts, and this is quite painful.

- Using free weights is more time consuming, because you have to add or take off weights for different exercises.

- There are some exercises, especially many leg exercises, which are much easier and more efficient when done on a machine.

- The correct movement is established for you with machines. If you make sure the machine is set correctly for your size and height, you're about 80% of the way to doing the exercise correctly.

- Machines do a better job of isolating muscles that are being worked. For people with injuries, machines allow a person to exercise without as much strain on injured body parts.

There are also a few exercises that I think are important which can only be done correctly with a machine (either home or gym).

The more you sweat in training, the less

you bleed in battle. Roman proverb

If you plan to work out at home, the whole decision of free weights versus machines becomes trickier. A machine costs a lot more than a few sets of dumbbells, and it takes up a lot of space. Because of its size and intrusiveness, a home weight machine will become a part of your life whether you use it or not. As you can guess, it isn't easy to pick up a machine that has a 150 pound weight stack so that you can vacuum under it.

Dumbbells are a nice thing to have in a home gym, but you will need several different weights. However, there are some pretty cool dumbbell products on the market today that let you quickly adjust the weight on a single set of dumbbells over a wide range using a sort of dial mechanism.

If you buy equipment for your home, check out the classified ads for used equipment. Many people buy fitness equipment, realize that they aren't going to use

 Machines aren't foolproof

Although machines help you to maintain proper form, they don't guarantee it. You still have to make sure that the machine is properly set up for your size and that you follow proper breathing and pace.

Choose the right equipment

When buying home equipment, stay away from one-dimensional exercise machines (for example, machines that only let you work your abs) that you see advertised on television or in magazines. Mail order equipment is generally overpriced and not as good quality as you get from a retail store. There are a couple of good general purpose machines sold by mail order but by and large you are better off getting a machine from a sporting goods or exercise equipment specialty retailer.

it and decide to sell it. If you buy from a disgruntled exerciser, negotiate the price – people often ask nearly full price with the rationale that the machine is "like new," but will bargain to get rid of that monstrosity that's collecting dust and reminding them of their failed vow to exercise.

Let's summarize this discussion about free weights versus machines so we can all get on with our lives. If you're a beginner and if you choose a gym, I suggest that you use machines until you become comfortable with the whole strength training scene. A strength training machine for your home gym is the ideal. But if you'd rather not take the financial plunge right away, you can start with some dumbbells of various weights ranging from 3 pounds to 15 pounds each for ladies and 10 pounds to 25 pounds each for men, a bench and a cardio machine of some kind.

Chapter Six

Ideas for scheduling your sessions

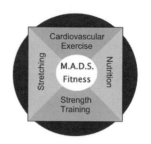

Remember in a previous chapter, we said that the ideal schedule is to work out three or four times a week with each workout consisting of a full body strength training workout combined with cardiovascular exercise?

Let the compromising begin!

I have used a three-or-four-times-a-week schedule pretty faithfully for the past many years, oftentimes working 10 or 12 hour days at my real job (unfortunately, being a fitness god doesn't pay consistently well) so it can be done. But there are a couple of drawbacks that I want to tell you about right up front.

First, a full body strength and cardio workout runs about 1-1/2 hours in length, depending on how many sets you do, how long you rest between sets, how much cardio you do, whether you do a lot of warm up or stretching and if you get involved in any chitchat between sets. That's a pretty big time commitment in one chunk and you have to plan your day around it.

Second, a full body workout can leave you pretty darn pooped out, especially when you start out. You may very well need an hour to lounge around after you finish a full workout.

I don't want you to get wrapped around the axle of doing things one way and one way only. The most important thing is that you get started on strength training and continue it. If you can't do it the ideal way, then let's figure out some good alternatives.

An "ideal" 3-times-a-week full body schedule looks like this:

DAY 1: FULL BODY STRENGTH AND CARDIO

DAY 2: DAY OFF (STRETCHING)

DAY 3: FULL BODY STRENGTH AND CARDIO

DAY 4: DAY OFF (STRETCHING)

DAY 5: FULL BODY STRENGTH AND CARDIO

DAY 6: DAY OFF (STRETCHING)

DAY 7: DAY OFF (OR WORK OUT - OPTIONAL)

Do you find it too hard to spend that much time at the gym? Here's an alternative that shortens your workout to about an hour:

DAY 1: UPPER BODY STRENGTH AND CARDIO

DAY 2: DAY OFF (STRETCHING)

DAY 3: LOWER BODY STRENGTH AND CARDIO

DAY 4: DAY OFF (STRETCHING)

DAY 5: UPPER BODY STRENGTH AND CARDIO

DAY 6: DAY OFF (STRETCHING)

DAY 7: LOWER BODY STRENGTH AND CARDIO

Do you want to get out of the gym in 45 minutes, or an hour at the very most? Or do you prefer to do your cardio at home and strength training at the gym (or vice versa)? If so, try this schedule:

DAY 1: UPPER BODY STRENGTH/STRETCHING

DAY 2: CARDIO/STRETCHING

DAY 3: LOWER BODY STRENGTH/STRETCHING

DAY 4: CARDIO/STRETCHING

DAY 5: UPPER/LOWER ALTERNATE BODY STRENGTH

DAY 6: CARDIO/STRETCHING

DAY 7: DAY OFF

Let's say you're a busy person who doesn't want to get home two hours later every night but can only get to the gym three days a week with maybe one of those days falling on the weekend. Try this schedule:

MON: UPPER BODY STRENGTH AND CARDIO

TUES: DAY OFF (STRETCHING)

WED: LOWER BODY STRENGTH AND CARDIO

THUR: DAY OFF (STRETCHING)

FRI: DAY OFF (STRETCHING)

SAT: FULL BODY STRENGTH AND CARDIO

SUN: DAY OFF (STRETCHING)

Remember the ingredients to a successful schedule that are listed below and then set up the schedule that works for you.

Speaking of making your schedule work for you, it's perfectly all right to shift between one schedule and another from week to week. Let's say this week you have some free time during the workweek and no special plans for the weekend. You plan a full body plus cardio workout for Monday, Wednesday, Friday and Sunday. The next week is going to be busy for you, since your spouse's Aunt Mabel is coming for her annual five-day (about 4-1/2 days too long) visit. That week, you sneak out of the house an hour early and get a half-workout in on Tuesday (remember you just did a full body workout Sunday so you should rest on Monday), Tuesday, Thursday and Friday. The following week, Monday and Tuesday are pretty clear but later in the week looks busy. You plan a full body workout on Monday, and try to squeeze two half-workouts in during the rest of the week.

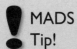 **MADS Tip!**   **However you decide to do it,**

a good schedule needs:

(a) At least one rest day between working the same area of the body

(b) Strength train every body area *at least* once per week (2 or 3 is better)

(c) Cardiovascular exercise at least three times per week

Chapter Seven

Sample strength training workouts

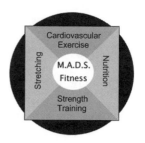

This chapter will give you some basic exercises, the real bread and butter exercises of strength training. You might not think it from looking at them, but weight lifters are a creative bunch, especially when it comes to self-torture. As a result, over the years many different variations of exercises have been devised.

Ideas for specific workouts

Here is the standard workout that I suggest for either men or women. It covers all body parts in a single workout. The main variation is the number of reps per set. Here is a general format:

Standard Full Body Workout

Exercise	Sets and Reps	Main muscle group
Leg Curl	3 sets of 10 reps	Legs - Quads
Hammie Curl	3 sets of 10 reps	Legs - Hamstrings
Leg Press/Squat	3 sets of 12 reps	Upper legs, glutes, hips
Calf Raise	3 sets of 12 reps	Calves
Chest Press	3 sets of 10 reps	Chest
Chest Flyes	3 sets of 10 reps	Chest

Seated Row	3 sets of 10 reps	Middle and lower back
Lat Pull-down	3 sets of 10 reps	Middle and upper back
Bicep Curl	3 sets of 10 reps	Arms - front of upper arm
Triceps Curl	3 sets of 10 reps	Arms - back of upper arm
Seated Press	3 sets of 10 reps	Shoulders
Shoulder Raise	3 sets of 10 reps	Shoulders
Ab Work	1 set of 30-60 reps	Tummy

Our MADS Body Area Workout has some nice advantages: It uses more calories so it's better for rapid weight loss, using lower weights results in less wear and tear on muscles, and there is a decreased chance of injury or strain. However, it also has some drawbacks. One is that the Body Area Workout tends to wear a person down over the long haul and you can fall into ruts where it's very hard to increase the amount of weight used. When that happens I switch to a split workout for a few weeks as a change of pace.

Split Workout using two workouts

Day One (focus on legs and chest):

Leg Curl	3 sets of 10 reps
Hammie Curl	3 sets of 10 reps
Leg Press	3 sets of 12 reps
Calf Raise	3 sets of 12 reps
Chest Press	3 sets of 10 reps

Chest Flyes	3 sets of 10 reps
Ab workout	1 set of 30-50 reps

Day Two (focus on back and arms)

Seated Row	3 sets of 10 reps
Lat Pull-down	3 sets of 10 reps
Biceps Curl	3 sets of 10 reps
Triceps Curl	3 sets of 10 reps
Seated Press	3 sets of 10 reps
Shoulder Raise	3 sets of 10 reps
Ab workout	1 set of 30-50 reps

Split Workout with three workouts

Day One (focus on legs):

Leg Curl	3 sets of 10 reps
Hammie Curl	3 sets of 10 reps
Leg Press	3 sets of 12 reps
Calf Raise	3 sets of 12 reps

Day Two (focus on core section):

Chest Press	3 sets of 10 reps
Chest Flyes	3 sets of 10 reps
Seated Row	3 sets of 10 reps
Lat Pull-down	3 sets of 10 reps

Ab workout   1 set of 30-50 reps

Day Three (focus on arms and shoulders):

Biceps Curl   3 sets of 10 reps

Triceps Curl   3 sets of 10 reps

Seated Press   3 sets of 10 reps

Shoulder Raise   3 sets of 10 reps

Ab workout   1 set of 30-50 reps

If you have an injury, or if exercising a particular body area is painful for any reason, you should adjust your routine to skip that area until it feels better.

Chapter Eight

Cardio Exercise Basics

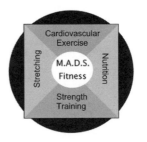

The second leg of our MADS fitness program is cardiovascular exercise. In strength training we've worked on building our muscles, but we haven't focused on the most important muscle of all: the heart. Our goal in cardiovascular exercise is to strengthen the heart, with a secondary goal of burning some additional calories to speed up weight loss or make maintaining our weight easier.

Running is the greatest metaphor for life, because

you get out of it what you put into it. Oprah Winfrey

Unlike strength training, CV exercise is pretty straightforward. In CV exercise we use the movement of our choice to increase the heart rates for several minutes at a time. Increasing the heart rate strengthens heart muscles and enhances our body's ability to process oxygen, both pretty good things in the big picture. If you add CV exercise to your schedule, you'll feel better, have more endurance and lessen your chance of a heart attack or stroke.

You and your heart rate

The secret to success in CV exercise is to increase your heart rate to a level that gives your heart a good workout. That heart rate level depends on your age and your physical condition. Once you hit your target heart rate (generally 50% to 85% of what your maximum heart rate is) you just have to work hard enough to maintain that level for at least 15 minutes.

To receive the complete benefit of CV exercise, it's important not to poop out too quickly. A super-fast heart rate for 5 minutes is not as good as having a heart rate in your desired CV range for 15 or 20 minutes.

Keeping track of your heart rate is really the only sure-fire way to know if you are working hard enough, or too hard. That means you will need to take your pulse periodically, which is hard enough when you're standing still, but we're going to make you do it while you're exercising to increase the degree of difficulty.

What are the ways to measure your heart rate?

(1) Take your own pulse. It's free! It's (not that) easy! Personally, I have a tough time doing this but if you'd like to try, here's how:

The best place to take your pulse is on your neck. Touch your left earlobe with your left middle finger. Now slide straight down an inch or so and you'll probably

Pacing yourself is especially important if you've been out of the exercise game for a while, so be sure to start slowly and work your way toward a higher heart rate. If you've had any health concerns in the past (especially hips, knees, ankles, heart or circulation problems) or are significantly overweight, you must get a doctor's OK before getting into any CV or strength training program.

find your jaw line. Now slide down another inch or so, move around a bit and you'll find a large artery. There may not be much of a pulse while you're sitting around reading, but when you're working out it will be stronger and easier to find.

I took up jogging to hear heavy

breathing again! Anonymous

When you take your pulse, use the timer on your CV equipment or look at a watch or clock. Count the number of beats for six seconds, and then multiply times ten. If you count 14 beats, your heart rate is 140 per minute. This isn't extremely precise, but you will get an estimate within 10 or so beats per minute.

(2) Use equipment with a heart monitor built in to it. If your club or home gym has equipment with heart monitoring capability, you can avoid measuring your heart rate yourself. Be forewarned, however, that these sensors (especially on health club equipment that gets used a lot) frequently end up out of whack so you may not get the most accurate of readings.

(3) Get a portable monitor. If you really dislike the idea of poking around your neck while exercising and your CV equipment doesn't have a heart monitor, buy a portable heart rate monitor that doubles as a wristwatch for as little as $70.

(4) Here is a less accurate but cheap and easy way. If you dislike both the idea of poking around your neck or spending upwards of $70, try using a "conversational pace" to monitor your heart rate. If you can talk and do your CV exercise at the same time, you aren't working too hard. If you can sing while exercising, you're probably not working hard enough (but you most certainly are annoying others around you). If you feel the need to stop and catch your breath at any point during CV exercise, you are definitely working too hard.

General guidelines for heart rates

The table shows estimated target heart rates for people of different ages. Look for the age category closest to yours, then read across to find your target heart rate. Your actual maximum and target may vary due to your weight and general physical condition. If you feel pain or serious shortness of breath, always stop exercising immediately. Some blood pressure medications lower the maximum heart rate and thus the target zone rate. If you're taking such medicine, call your physician for advice on your target heart rate.

Age	Target (50-85 % of max)	Maximum (100 %)
40 years	90–153 beats/minute	180 beats/minute
45 years	88–149 beats/minute	175 beats/minute
50 years	85–145 beats/minute	170 beats/minute
55 years	83–140 beats/minute	165 beats/minute
60 years	80–136 beats/minute	160 beats/minute
65 years	78–132 beats/minute	155 beats/minute
70 years	75–128 beats/minute	150 beats/minute
Source: American Heart Association		

You want your heart rate to be in the target range for several minutes, but it doesn't have to be that high for the entire time you exercise. It takes a few minutes to warm up, and you'll start winding down the intensity with a few minutes remaining in your allotted time. Your actual heart rate will typically look something like this, assuming a 20 minute cardio workout:

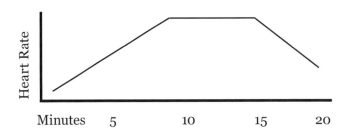

After you get a feel for how your heart rate responds to exercise and when it's within the desired range, you will likely cut way back on how often you check your heart rate. As you get into exercising regularly, you'll become pretty good at guessing where your heart rate is at.

If it gives you peace of mind to use a monitoring device, or your doctor suggests that you keep careful tabs on your heart rate, then by all means do so. If I'm using a machine that has heart monitoring capability, I generally check my heart rate a few times while I'm exercising. But as I've gotten more experienced, I've become better at estimating my heart rate by how I feel.

Chapter Nine

Getting on
track with CV

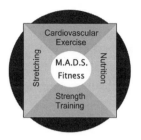

When starting a CV exercise program, we take the same approach as we do with strength training. Use the first few workouts to get the feel for the exercise you are doing. Maintain a comfortable pace and don't push it too hard.

If you're up to it on your third or fourth CV workout, aim for the lowest part of your target heart rate range (50%). Then gradually build up to about 75% over the next four weeks.

How fast you increase the workload is up to you. Do what your body tells you, but try to gradually increase your workload by increasing some combination of: (1) your pace, (2) the length of time that you work out or (3) the resistance.

Choose the CV exercise that's right for you

The fitness industry has devised several torture...oops, I mean helpful machines to assist you in increasing your heart rate. If none of those suit you, there are a other ways to get CV exercise that are free of charge and probably close by.

Common types of CV equipment include:

Treadmill: The old standby in the CV world is still the treadmill. Treadmills offer two types of resistance: (1) speed at which the belt travels, and (2) incline of the base. The faster you travel and the steeper the incline, the greater your workload will be.

Treadmills are easy to use for beginners and usually offer a "softer" surface than pavement, so they are easier on your joints than walking on the sidewalk. You also have precise control over the speed and incline. Although they are considerably easier on knees and hips than concrete, treadmills can still be rough on people with joint problems.

Stepper: There are different variations of steppers, also called stair climbers. Whatever their name, they basically imitate the motion of climbing stairs. You can usually set the resistance and control the speed at which you move.

Steppers are easier on the joints than climbing actual steps. They provide an intense exercise that gets your heart rate going fast in a short period. The leg muscles, especially quads and calves, get a strengthening workout while your heart gets a cardio workout.

MADS Tip!

CV Machine Buying Tip

If you're buying CV equipment, one of the biggest factors in the price is the electronic features on a particular model. Features like the resistance adjusting automatically to your heartrate and built-in programs that allow you to set up different workout profiles tend to add quite a bit onto the price. Carefully weigh the features versus the value that you think you'll get from them before you pop for higher end electronics.

Steppers are difficult for beginners so I suggest starting with a treadmill, elliptical trainer or stationary bike for a few months and, if you want, throwing in a stepper after that for the sake of variety.

Elliptical trainer: On elliptical trainers, you place your feet on pads and then move them in a sort of gliding or cross-country skiing motion. The pads are on tracks that guide your feet forward and back, and your feet end up moving in sort of an elliptical (Attention Stoughton, Wisconsin readers: elliptical is kind of like an oval) shape, hence the name. Most machines let you adjust both the resistance and incline, and also vary your speed.

Elliptical trainers are easier on the hips and knees than treadmills. I find elliptical trainers the most enjoyable form of cardio exercise, but that's personal preference as much as anything else.

> *You have to believe in you because*
> *sometimes that's the only person who*
> *does believe in your success.* Tim Blixseth

The biggest drawback of elliptical trainers is that they can be a little tricky for beginners to use. It's somewhat intimidating to have to step up a bit to get to the pads, and elliptical trainers require a basic presence of mind to keep your balance while you're exercising. But they aren't as difficult as they seem, and most people get the hang of using them pretty quickly. For home gyms, elliptical trainers are typically the most expensive CV machine option.

Rower: Rowing machines drift in and out of popularity in the fitness world. There are various shapes and sizes on the market.

Rowers give an upper body as well as lower body workout because you pull with your arms and push with your legs while you row. Since we are already hitting the rest of our body with strength training, rowing for cardio exercise is above and beyond the call of duty. Those with back problems should obviously be careful about rowing. That said, if your back is up to it and you enjoy rowing (as many people do) please don't hesitate to row, row and then row some more.

Stationary bicycle: These days there are two basic forms of stationary bike: (1) upright and (2) seated. Upright bikes put you in the position you associate most with riding an actual bicycle; sitting more or less upright on a saddle with the pedals directly below you. On a seated bike, you are in something resembling a chair, with the pedals in front of you. Many people feel that seated bikes offer a lot easier experience for your back and the rest of your upper body, while an upright bike takes a bit more effort but better simulates riding a real bicycle. I don't have a preference and use both types occasionally.

Bicycles typically offer the lowest impact form of cardio exercise available on a machine. A bike can be especially helpful when you have a sore leg muscle or achy Achilles tendon because you can have a decent cardio exercise without aggravating the injury. A bicycle allows you to vary the resistance and speed to customize your workout.

Home cardio equipment

If you're thinking of equipment for your home, you have an important decision ahead of you. At a gym, you're able to move at a whim from a bike to a treadmill to an elliptical trainer – not so at home where you probably have space and dollars to buy only one of the above. You have one shot at making the right decision, little missy, so it better be a good one.

All of the pluses and minuses we just mentioned apply to home equipment, but you also need to consider size and bulk of the equipment as well as its reliability.

No matter how hard manufacturers try, a quality piece of CV equipment is going to be heavy and pretty big. Sure, there are fold-up treadmills and the like, but even folded up, a good treadmill takes up some room.

My lovely wife, The Bride-of-Self-Proclaimed-Fitness-Expert, prefers to do her cardio in the comfort of our home, and the treadmill is her weapon of choice in the battle to stay in shape. So I have intimate experience with the disadvantages of home exercise equipment. A decent treadmill is bulky and really heavy. I think of the treadmill's trip down the basement steps as a one-way journey.

The other thing I've found is that cardio exercise equipment has parts that have to be replaced now and then. Unless you're eager to get a hernia, it's not practical to take the equipment to a repair shop. So your options are to buy the parts and become a repair expert, or call a repair person to make a house call. If you're looking for a new career, think about being a home exercise equipment repair person. There aren't many of them, they certainly don't work overtime, and judging from how much they charge, they make more than a brain surgeon.

If reliability was my main concern for home equipment, I would choose stationary bikes as most reliable, followed by rowing machines, then by treadmills, and in last place, elliptical trainers. For decent quality home equipment that is used regularly, I would anticipate a useful life five to seven years and I would budget 30% to 40% of the up-front cost of the equipment for repairs that will be needed over the life of the equipment.

CV exercise without machines

You don't necessarily have to use a machine to get a CV workout. There are a number of machine-free options for CV exercise. Here are the most common:

Walking: If you've been sitting on your duff for a few years and want to get back into the game, walking is the ideal way to start. All you need is a watch and your own two feet inserted into a comfy pair of sneakers or walking shoes. Start out with a distance you feel comfortable with and a leisurely walking pace, then gradually increase the pace and distance as you get into better shape. Stick with walking for a few months and you may need additional challenge; at that time you can decide to use a treadmill or other machine.

> *If walking is so good for you, then why does my*
> *mailman look like Jabba the Hut?* Anonymous

The biggest mistake people make in walking for CV exercise is not walking fast enough. You should be able to hold a conversation while walking, but you should try to find the pace at which conversation becomes difficult, then back off a bit.

If you suffer from knee, hip, heart, circulatory or back problems I really, really want you to seek the advice of your doctor before choosing the type of CV exercise you undertake, including walking.

Jogging: This is basically a more intense form of walking. If walking is your preferred CV exercise, you may eventually end up jogging as you get in better shape in order to reach your desired heart rate.

For middle-agers, the biggest drawback to jogging is that it results in your various body parts getting jolted and bounced around, which isn't something to take lightly. A couple of years ago, I decided to take up running for my CV exercise as a change of pace and a month later ended up having surgery to repair a detached retina. Coincidence or cause-and-effect? I'll never know for sure, but I blame the bouncing that running put my body through.

 MADS Tip!

Here is a way to guesstimate the intensity of your walking:

Low intensity: Like window shopping in the mall.

Low-Medium intensity: Like you're a bit late to meet a friend.

Medium-High intensity: Like you're a bit late to meet your boss.

High intensity: Like your airplane is boarding without you.

My personal suspicions about my eyeball aside, it's a well-accepted fact that jogging is tougher on knees, ankles, feet, lower back and hips than other forms of CV exercise, and I generally do not recommend it.

Stair climbing: This is not for the faint of heart or out-of-shape, because stairs can be a challenge. If you're just getting started, I would avoid stair climbing and stick to walking, biking or exercise machines. If you are the one person reading this book who enjoys stair climbing as a form of exercise, it is something you could add into your routine, but not for the first couple of months.

> *If it weren't for the fact that the TV set and the*
>
> *refrigerator are so far apart,*
>
> *I wouldn't get any exercise at all!* Unknown

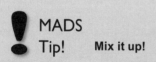

MADS Tip!   **Mix it up!**

There's certainly nothing wrong with mixing things up and experimenting with several types of exercise. You may decide to bike once a week, walk a few times, and swim once a week. Or maybe you prefer a couple days a week of CV work in a gym and a couple of days outdoors.

Swimming: A lot of people prefer swimming as their favorite CV exercise. Swimming laps is great exercise and offers the benefit of being a lot easier on your knees and hips than most other alternatives. We must differentiate between splashing around in the water and swimming. To get any CV benefit, you should swim laps non-stop for at least 15 to 20 minutes.

Bicycling: If the weather's nice and you enjoy the outdoors, biking can be a really fun way to get your CV workout. Like walking, the main thing to pay attention to is your pace. A leisurely bike ride might be relaxing and enjoyable, but it isn't CV exercise. You need to work hard enough to get your heart rate into the desired range for at least 15 to 20 minutes. Some people find biking to be much easier on the back, knees, hips and feet than jogging or walking.

Aerobics, Spinning, kick boxing and other group CV

If you're a social type and enjoy exercising with others, you may want to consider joining a gym and participating in group fitness classes. If you're interested in classes and don't belong to a gym yet, be sure to carefully examine the schedule of classes before you commit to joining. Some health clubs have extensive CV classes and some have little or nothing offered.

Group exercise can be a lot of fun and provides variety for CV exercise. There are literally hundreds of different group CV activities, ranging from simple aerobic dance to martial arts to stationary biking and many more.

Making CV exercise part of your overall fitness

There are countless ways to combine CV into your overall fitness program, but the main decision boils down to either (a) doing cardio and strength training in the same session, or (b) doing strength training and cardio on separate days.

Some studies indicate that doing strength training and cardio in one session uses more calories than if done separately. But the advantage isn't huge, so that isn't a reason to combine cardio with strength training if it's not otherwise convenient. Remember, your main goal is to make exercise a part of your life, so making your program one you can live with is always the overriding factor.

Generally, the cardio portion of a workout is 25 to 35 minutes. That includes an exercise time of 20 to 30 minutes plus about 5 minutes to cool down. If you're already spending close to an hour on strength training, your workout is now pushing 1-1/2 hours long. One consideration is whether you have that much time to spend in one chunk. On the flip side, if you combine cardio and strength training, you can get away with working out three or four times per week.

I get my exercise acting as a pallbearer to my

friends who never exercised. Anonymous

Should you decide to use your non-strength training days for cardio, you will be exercising six days a week, but on the other hand, your workouts will be shorter in length. Instead of three or four workouts of 75 to 90 minutes, you'll be doing six workouts of about 45 to 60 minutes.

In case you glossed over it, the strength training section in this book has a bunch of sample schedules including strength training and CV exercise that reflect the combinations we just talked about.

Keep things challenging

As we said at the start of this chapter, our MADS philosophy of always trying to increase the amount of work we do also applies to CV exercise. There are three variables that we can change to increase our cardiovascular workload: (1) length of time we do it, (2) amount of resistance, and (3) speed or pace.

The idea is to slowly increase one or more of these factors over a number of weeks and months. When you are first getting started with a CV routine, you may increase one or more of the factors once a week. But as you get more experienced you will find that increases don't come as easily, maybe only once a month.

Increasing the length of time you do cardio exercise can only get you so far (if you are walking for exercise, there was no pun intended), because eventually you'll reach the point where you can't set aside the time required to keep exercising longer and longer. I have seen a number of people at the gym who spend an hour or more on a treadmill. In my opinion, that goes far beyond the point of diminishing returns in terms of the heart benefits received.

If you are spending so much time on the treadmill that you feel like a hamster on a wheel, try shortening the time you spend and increase the resistance or speed. Instead of walking for a longer time, try to go one-tenth of a mile further in the same time period. If that doesn't work for you, then set the resistance a notch higher or crank up the incline a little bit.

Grandma started walking for her health

when she was 60. Now she's 62 and

we don't know where the heck she is! Unknown

Did I make it clear that I think cardio sessions over 30 minutes are a waste of time when it comes to heart health? Besides not being more beneficial to your heart, longer CV sessions put more wear and tear on your knees, hips and ankles. For example, I average about 170 strides per minute on an elliptical trainer. That means for every 10 minutes extra that I exercise, I am taking 1,700 more strides. At four times a week over the course of a year, that's 353,000 additional times my hips and knees have flexed – that's a lot of extra wear and tear!

The point is, don't over-do it. Certainly you should do enough cardio to get the heart benefits you're looking for, but don't get carried away and waste hours on CV that you could be spending on something else.

There's a difference between CV exercise and exercising with the goal of weight loss. If your goal is to burn calories, there *is* a benefit to spending more time on a treadmill. You will burn more calories the longer you do it. The key difference is that for weight loss exercise, you don't have to keep your heart rate at the same elevated level as you do in CV exercise, so you can use a slower pace.

How much CV exercise is the right amount?

Now that I've told you not to spend too much time on CV, how much is the right amount? The so-called experts say (and as a self-proclaimed expert, I concur with my esteemed, self-proclaimed colleagues) to get any health benefit, you need to do a minimum of 15 to 20 minutes of cardio, 3 to 4 times a week. Some studies say that you get increasing benefit from up to 30 minutes of cardio per session. So, anywhere between 15 minutes and 30 minutes is a good, beneficial cardio session. How much cardio you decide to do depends on your fitness goals and how much time you have on your hands.

Over the years, I have come up with little mental tricks to make CV exercise more challenging. You are welcome to devise your own, but here are some ideas:

- Many pieces of CV equipment have a calorie calculator built in. I often use the calorie count as my goal – for instance, I try to burn off 300 calories in 20 minutes. As I go along, I keep my mind occupied trying to figure out if I'm on pace to hit my goal: How many calories per minute am I using? Will my current pace get me to my goal?

- Machines also display distance traveled. I will often set a distance goal for my workout and try to achieve that in a set period of time. For example, I may shoot for two miles in 20 minutes. Again, you can keep yourself busy by trying to figure out if you're on pace to reach your goal.

One thing that I *don't* do during CV exercise is read a book or magazine. I find it impossible to push myself as hard as I need to while simultaneously focusing on reading something. I also am incapable of doing two things at once without losing my balance and falling off whatever CV machine I am on, which is the same reason I only chew gum while seated. I do watch TV while doing CV since it's easy to do that and still pay attention to the exercise.

> *I like long walks, especially when they are taken by*
> *people who annoy me.* Fred A. Allen

To get into better and better shape, get an idea of what your current level of performance is and then try to improve it by setting slightly higher goals. Playing "games" is a way to help you set goals so that you continually increase your CV workload in a fun way.

If your goal is weight loss, you may find it beneficial to increase your cardio sessions to four to six times per week. If you're looking to strengthen your heart and lessen your risk of heart attack and stroke, three to four times a week should be enough to do the trick.

Chapter Ten

The MADS Nutrition Plan

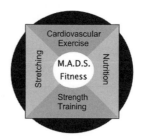

I recently came up with a unique and very effective diet plan. The plan I devised is based on a little-known recipe for "fly wing soup" that I discovered on a trip to the remote island of Pago Pago. I noticed that the villagers there were all very thin, and I learned that the primary staple of their diet was a soup made from the wings of a species of fly that inhabit their island. And then I woke up…

Whew! I'm glad that was only a dream. But when you look at the crazy nutrition plans out there today, fly wing soup isn't awfully far out of line.

It's easy to lose weight. Just shut your pie hole and get on a treadmill.

MJ Kelli, Florida radio personality

MADS is just the opposite of those crazy diet plans. Here is the basis for the MADS nutrition plan: (1) choose the right kinds of foods, (2) eat moderate portions and (3) exercise in order to burn up some calories. If you do these three things you will lose weight.

Not exactly out there on the fringe, huh? But in the end, this approach is the only one that actually works. In spite of what the TV infomercials and advertisements say, there is no magic way to lose weight. There are no secret foods or drinks that will double your metabolism. There are no diet pills, drinks or drugs that guarantee successful weight loss. All the popular fad diets – Subway, Atkins, South Beach and the rest – work for one simple reason: like any other diet that works, they involve ultimately reducing the number of calories that you eat relative to the calories that your body uses.

What we'll do is lay out an easy to follow plan to lose weight, or maintain your current weight if that's what you want to do.

The beauty of the MADS nutrition plan is its flexibility. You can set the plan up to help you reach your individual goal.

Losing weight – nutrition basics

I'm going to focus on you folks who would like to lose a few pounds, since every study I've seen recently says you are in the majority. Over 60% of adults in the United States are now considered overweight, and nearly half of those people fit into the "obese" category (and *don't* fit into their clothes).

Why does a person become overweight? Think of your body as an engine. Like an engine, you need fuel to run. Even when you are snoozing in an easy chair, your body is using fuel for necessary things like breathing, keeping your heart beating and everything else your body does for you that you thanklessly take for granted, being the ungrateful bum that you are. The fuel your body needs to operate comes from the food you eat. But what happens when a person takes in more fuel than their body needs? The human body has a way to take care of that – it converts the extra food energy into fat, which the body stores away – unfortunately for you and me, it stores the fat in highly visible places.

Why you shouldn't feel guilty about that excess weight

Many people are burdened not only with extra pounds, but also with guilt. That guilt in turn can make a person more likely to turn to food for solace, leading to even more guilt, which in turn leads to more eating, which increases guilt yet again which causes more eating...and the vicious circle goes on and on.

I'm here to tell you that, if you're overweight, there is no reason in the world to feel guilty about it. Becoming overweight is a perfectly natural response to living in today's modern world, and I'm going to explain why.

The older you get the harder it is to lose weight,

because by then your body and

your fat have become good friends. Anonymous

The story begins a long time ago, when cavemen lurched around the earth. As you can imagine, being a caveman was no picnic. Oh sure, there were good times when a lost wooly mammoth happened by and the caveman-of-the-house got lucky with his slingshot. Then it was fine dining for a few days. But much of the time, our cavemen ancestors resorted to foraging for berries and grains, usually finding just enough food to get by.

Even back then, the human body was highly adaptable. The body adapted to the caveman's "feast or famine" lifestyle by becoming very efficient at converting excess woolly mammoth calories into fat, then storing the fat away to be used during lean times, when roots and berries were the only items on the menu.

In today's society, most people don't live a feast or famine lifestyle. In fact most lifestyles today are best described as "feast or feast more." Not only do we have plenty of food, but we are blessed with an endless supply of calorie-dense, delicious food that our ancestor cavemen never even dreamed about. Excuse me a minute, I have to take a break...OK, I'm back – let me just wipe those Twinkie® crumbs off my keyboard. Now, where was I?

! MADS Tip!

Some foods for a healthier heart

Grape juice: Red wine gets all the publicity, but the heart-healthiness of wine comes from red or purple grapes, so drinking grape juice provides the benefits without having to get plowed every night.

Salmon: Bears eat a lot of salmon. Have you ever seen a bear have a heart attack? Neither have I, but that's beside the point. Salmon has a lot of omega-3 fatty acids, which have been found to reduce heart attack risk.

Spinach: Spinach is one of the better things you can yank out of the ground, wash the sand off of, and eat. Lots better than worms, for one. Spinach has folate, which has been shown to reduce some heart-nasty stuff in your blood called homocysteine.

Sweet potatoes: These orange monstrosities qualify as one of our heart-healthy foods because of their fiber, antioxidant levels, and vitamin content.

Unfortunately for us, our bodies still think we live in a "feast or famine" world, so our bodies merrily turn every stinking extra calorie that we eat into fat (not that I'm bitter about it). Since we rarely find ourselves in famine situations in modern society, the extra fat just keeps building up.

There are some additional factors at work as well. Many foods today have some powerful fat-builders that even our parents didn't have working against them. Two big culprits are high fructose corn sweetener and trans fats. We'll discuss these in more detail in a while.

> *The way you think, the way you behave, the way you eat,*
>
> *can influence your life by 30 to 50 years.* Deepak Chopra

The bottom line is this: If you're overweight and feeling guilty about it, get with the American way and blame somebody else for your problems! Feel free to spread the blame among your ancestors, those big food processing corporations and while we're at it, we may as well blame life in general.

Seriously, if you're overweight, you need to stop feeling guilty and realize that it's the result of the natural order of evolution combined with some flaws in today's nutritional marketplace. So I want you to do this right now: stop feeling guilty and start thinking of how you're going to overcome these obstacles.

Does your food make the grade?

What we do in MADS is give each food a letter grade, just like in school. Remember back in school when your folks told you to keep away from all the "bad kids" and hang out with the good kids that studied hard and got good grades? If you're like me, you not only didn't heed that advice, but ended up (to borrow a line from singer Jimmy Buffet) being one of the people your parents warned you about. If you didn't listen to mom and dad back then, here's your chance to get it right this time by hanging out with the right foods.

The rules are simple:

(1) Choose foods from the A-list and B-list whenever possible. With the exception of meat, fish, brown rice and sweet potatoes, you can eat as much of the A-list foods as you'd like, and reasonable amounts of the B-list foods. The foods on the A-list are generally full of good things and low in calories. B-list foods offer positives but have drawbacks – some are calorie-dense, others are slightly high in fats.

(2) Eat C-list foods in limited amounts. Our C-list items aren't horrible for you, but they won't do much good for you, either.

(3) You don't have to completely eliminate D-list foods, but try to keep them to a minimum. The only D-list foods you should have on a semi-regular basis are breads. Limit your eating of breads to one serving, and not every day. The non-bread D-list foods should be eaten minimally, if at all.

(4) Avoid foods from the F-list, except on rare occasions. These foods can be a very small and very infrequent part of your diet, but definitely not a day-to-day indulgence.

A-foods list

Berries

Apples and pears

Other fruits and vegetables

Green tea

Carrots

Broccoli

Cauliflower

Chicken and turkey breast

Soups (not creamy or cheesy and easy on the crackers)

Salmon, tuna and other fish (broiled or baked, canned tuna is OK)

Fat-free milk

Green beans and similar beans

Kidney beans, black beans and pinto beans

Oatmeal

Spinach

Boston, Romaine or Iceberg lettuce

Ground turkey (compare labels, all are not equal)

Sweet potatoes

Brown rice (limit 1 cup cooked per day)

B-foods list

Nuts and peanut butter (watch your portions on these)

Low fat cheeses (limit 1 serving daily)

Yogurt (preferably low fat and sugar free)

White potatoes (baked only)

Citrus fruits (oranges and grapefruit)

Citrus fruit juices (no sugar added)

Some breakfast cereals (low sugar, high fiber)

Lean beef and pork

Brown, black and white teas

Eggs (boiled or poached)

Low calorie and low fat salad dressings (as desired)

Cooking spray and pump liquid margarine

C-foods list

Coffee and traditional tea

Crisp bacon

Starches: White rice, corn and peas

Baked snacks, pretzels, Quakes® brand snacks and rice cakes

Lean cold cuts (turkey and chicken, low sodium if possible)

Diet soft drinks

D-foods list

Breads, rolls and bagels

High fat cheeses

Whole ice cream

Sausage and hot dogs

Fried fish

Beer and wine

Low fat sherbet and ice cream

F-foods list

Donuts, pastries and muffins

Cookies and cakes

Fast food menu items (except salads)

French fries

Traditional snack foods (regular potato chips, etc.)

Sugar (non-diet) soft drinks

Most fruit juices (other than citrus and grape juice)

Pickled or smoked meats and sausage

High fat cold cuts (bologna, salami, etc.)

Alcoholic beverages other than beer and wine

Candy and chocolate

Confessions of an oatmeal addict

I've eaten so much oatmeal in the past decade that I should get a thank you card each year from Quaker Oats. A typical week will find me eating oatmeal for breakfast at least five days, usually six days. My dogs have developed a sense of entitlement about having a couple of tablespoons of cooked oatmeal with their regular breakfast.

Although everyone recognizes the health benefits, oatmeal has gotten a bad rap. Oatmeal's image of being blah-tasting mush was created by cooks with little imagination. Think of oatmeal as kind of like a baked potato – it isn't that great all by itself but when you add some flavor it can be really (well, sort of) delicious.

But back to the health benefits side of things. Oatmeal is rich in the kind of fiber that acts like a vacuum to suck up bad cholesterol in your digestive system before it gets absorbed. The fiber keeps things moving, if you get my drift, which lowers your risk of colon cancer. Another benefit is that if you eat oatmeal for breakfast, chances are it's replacing something less healthy like bacon and eggs.

Here are your favorite author's tips for making oatmeal a healthy, easy and yummy part of your diet:

- Use quick oats, which are just as healthy as regular oats. A bowl of quick oats cooks in 90 seconds in the microwave (and boils over in about 120).

- Avoid the pre-packaged envelopes. They not only cost a lot more, but they are loaded with salt and sugar. Even the plain flavor contains a huge amount of salt. Stick with bulk oatmeal, the kind sold in canisters. If you must use flavored packages, before cooking, mix one-half of a flavored package with one-third cup of quick oats from a canister. You'll still have great-tasting oatmeal with one-half the sodium and sugar.

• Keep a small measuring cup right inside the canister, so you have it handy to measure your oats. I usually guesstimate the amount of water.

• Add just a pinch of salt in making your oatmeal. Add fat-free milk after cooking to get the consistency you prefer.

• To keep your oats low-cal, use an artificial sweetener. I use a couple of the blue or the yellow packets, but mix it with one tablespoon of sugar or honey to make it more filling. Don't worry about how much artificial sweetener you use – the idea is to make your oatmeal the way you like it.

Here are some ideas of stuff to add to your oatmeal:

MADS Tip!

Blueberries	Raisins	Dried or canned fruit	
Strawberries	Diced apple	Pumpkin pie mix	Applesauce
Bananas	Cinnamon	Vanilla	Peaches

Check out a company called Penzey's Spices (www.Penzeys.com) for top notch cinnamon – it costs a few cents more per serving but it is head and shoulders above the grocery store variety. My favorites are the Vietnamese Cassia or Chinese Cassia. Penzey's also sells several kinds of vanilla that are amazing.

Fiber: Here today, gone tomorrow

One of the biggest issues that nutritionists have with our modern diet is that it lacks enough fiber. Fiber is good, because it keeps food moving through the old pipes. I don't know about you, but I wish to avoid ending up like my grandmother, whose favorite subject of conversation was what she politely referred to as her "bowel movements." The best way to keep things on an even keel in that department is to eat plenty of fiber.

> *The second day of a diet is always*
>
> *easier than the first. By the second day*
>
> *you're off it.* Jackie Gleason

The average person eats about 15 grams of fiber a day; that's one-half of the 30-plus grams recommended by people who know more than me or you. There are plenty of ways to get your 30 grams of fiber per day. For instance, a single serving of oatmeal has at least 4 grams of fiber. Pears and apples are also great sources of fiber, but so are many other fruits. Dried fruits are loaded with fiber – for instance just a quarter cup of dried apricots has 11 grams. Dried fruits are calorie dense, so don't eat too many of them. There are some cereals that are also good sources of fiber. You may find it difficult to choke down Kellogg's All Bran® straight, but why not mix a quarter cup of it with another kind of cereal that you do like? A quarter cup of Kellogg's All Bran® is only 40 calories but packs a 5-gram punch of fiber.

A dietary villain

According to the researchers that keep track of the number of overweight citizens (if that was your job, how would you explain it to people?) if the U.S. were wearing pants, those trousers would be splitting at the seams. As a country, America has been packing on the pounds like there's no tomorrow. Almost two-thirds of Americans are now classified as overweight, up from less than one-quarter in the late 1980s. About one-third of the U.S. population falls (look out below!) into the obese category.

That weight gain is in spite of the ever-increasing number of people who are trying to lose weight. People are spending more money and trying harder than ever to keep weight off, yet they find themselves putting on the pounds at a faster rate than ever before.

There are lots of possible reasons for this trend. The simplest is that we are bombarded with advertising for highly processed foods, and most people have the money to indulge our food whims.

You can't lose weight by talking about it. You have to

keep your mouth shut! Anonymous

But as I mentioned earlier, there is another culprit at least partly responsible for this trend: High Fructose Corn Sweetener (HFCS). The weight gain that has happened to our country as a whole is highly correlated to the growth of HFCS as a food ingredient.

What is High Fructose Corn Sweetener? Without getting too scientific, it's a concentrated (20 times sweeter than table sugar) product made from corn. HFCS is cheaper to produce than cane or beet sugar, it can be mixed more easily with other foods during manufacturing, and it has a longer shelf life. That has made HFCS a popular product with food manufacturers, and it has swept into many, many foods on store shelves. And not just the foods you'd expect, like donuts and soft drinks. HFCS can be found in fruit juices, dairy products and even bread.

The *American Journal of Clinical Nutrition* (April 2004) said the intake of HFCS in the U.S. increased by 1,000% between 1970 and 1990. Another way to look at the increase is to compare how much HFCS we ate in 1960 (zero pounds per person, since it hadn't been developed yet) with how much HFCS the average person ate in 2001 – a whopping 63 pounds!

Here's another statistic that should scare you, this one courtesy of "Nourishing Traditions" by Sally Fallon and Mary Enig: In 1994 (not that long ago – I still have some socks I bought that year), sugars made up 19% of the calories Americans consumed. In 2006, the percentage of calories from sugars was 25%.

If HFCS is the problem, what's the solution? Try to avoid it, which is easier said than done. Many packaged foods have HFCS, but by reading nutritional labels you can catch the worst offenders. Look for "fructose," "corn sweetener," or any similar words in the first few ingredients. By law, ingredients must be listed in the order of the content by weight, so the first items listed are usually the most important.

Omega-3 fats: They're not a fish story

If you look back over history at the typical human diet, the amount of omega-3 fats (considered a "good fat") in American diets has declined since the early 1900s while saturated fats, omega-6 fats and trans fats (all bad fats) are a larger percentage of diets.

Some scientists say omega-3 fats could be helpful for preventing a wide range of health problems including heart attacks, strokes, Alzheimer's disease, arthritis, depression and cancer.

To be fair, there are two sides to this fish story. The Food and Nutrition Board and the U.S. Food and Drug Administration have ignored or downplayed omega-3's benefits. My opinion is that there is enough medical opinion and anecdotal evidence (anecdotal evidence is a fancy way of saying, "A friend of my friend told her brother that...") in favor of omega-3 fats, that you should consider making them a part of your diet.

Supporters say that omega-3 fats increase brain function and prevention of Alzheimer's disease. About 20% of our brains are made up of DHA, one kind of omega-3 fat, so it stands to reason that eating DHA helps the brain. Omega-3 backers also claim reduced inflammation in arteries. Many doctors say that an inflammation process is what eventually leads to heart attack and stroke. In Europe, a prescription drug called Omacor is often used to treat cardiac patients. Omacor is – you guessed it – highly purified DHA and EPA, two ingredients of omega-3 fats.

There are two ways to get omega-3 fats: (1) eat certain types of fish that are rich in omega-3 fats, or (2) take supplements containing omega-3 fats. Personally, I do both because it's almost impossible to ensure you'll get an adequate amount through eating fish alone.   *(Continued)*

The most common fish sources of omega-3 fats are salmon, mackerel, tuna and sardines. The problem with eating large amounts of fish these days is that a lot of fish (especially farm-raised fish) contains higher levels of mercury and other contaminants than in the past. That's not bad if you eat fish less than once a week and minimize eating of farm-raised fish. But to get the amount of omega-3 fats you need, you should eat fish twice a week or more. If you've compared the price of wild salmon to farm-raised salmon you are aware that it is easy to go to the poorhouse buying wild salmon. To paraphrase the saying, "Give a man a fish and he'll eat for a day. Teach a man to shop for wild salmon and he'll be broke in a week."

So go ahead and eat salmon (or other cold water fish like good old tuna) once in a while. But buy a good fish oil supplement as your main source of omega-3 fats. Be sure to buy a supplement made from fish oil, not flaxseed (although I also eat flaxseed) or algae oil (would you want to eat algae oil anyway?). Only fish oil contains both EPA and DHA, two abbreviations for important-sounding names of the critical acids that make up omega-3 fat.

When you shop for a fish oil supplement, ignore the total milligrams (mg) and look on the label for how much EPA and DHA each capsule contains. You want to take in at least 500 mg per day of combined EPA and DHA. Most capsules come in a ratio of EPA to DHA of 3:2, for example 300 mg of EPA and 200 mg of DHA. You can buy liquid or capsules, the choice is yours.

Important: If you are on blood thinners, ask your doctor about the best dosage for you before you start taking omega-3 supplements.

! MADS Tip!

Better yet, stick to the A and B-list foods shown above, which should have little or no HFCS. The only A and B foods you need to check labels on are peanut butter, yogurt and breakfast cereals – look for brands that don't have HFCS terms among the first few ingredients.

To get rid of fat you have to know your fats

You've probably heard that there are "good" fats and "bad" fats.

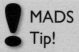

MADS Tip!

How can you keep track of the percentage of calories from fat? Look at the labels on the foods you eat, which now are required to display the percentage of calories from fat. If a serving has 200 calories total and 60 calories from fat, that is 30%. If you eat 10 servings, what percentage of calories come from fat? Still 30% but that was a trick question because you shouldn't be eating 10 servings of anything in one sitting, you silly goose.

What's the deal with that? Simply stated, there are three kinds of fats that are naturally occurring in food: saturated, monounsaturated, and polyunsaturated. There's also additional one category of fat that is man-made, and that is the dreaded *trans fat.*

Is fat bad? Not necessarily. Eaten in moderation, the right kinds of fats are a necessary and valuable part of a person's diet. The problem with fat comes in when we eat fat in excess instead of moderation and eat the wrong kind of fats.

The solution is simple: Eat fats in moderation (no more than 30% of your total calories should come from fat) and try to stick to the best fats, which are the poly-

MADS
Tip!   **Recognizing and avoiding bad fats**

• Check the nutritional label for type and amount of fat in the food you eat. Avoid foods that are high in saturated fats, trans fats, or have the words "hydrogenated" or "partially hydrogenated" in the ingredients.

• When you buy cooking oil, always go for mono-or-poly-fat oils like olive oil, soybean oil, corn oil and sunflower oil.

• Generally, fats that are hard at room temperature or in the fridge are bad, and ones that are soft or liquid at room temperature are good. Buy soft margarine in tub or spray form instead of sticks, butter, lard or solid shortening.

• Eat more chicken, turkey, fish and lean pork. Trim off visible fat when eating red meat. Don't eat too much poultry skin, as most of the fat content in chicken and turkey is in that part.

• Be careful when dining out. The Internet has a lot of information regarding quick service chain foods (see www.MADSfitness.com for links). In sit-down restaurants, have food prepared in a low-fat manner – avoid deep fried and pan fried foods as well as cream sauces. Be a pain in the rear, and ask the waiter to make sure the kitchen avoids smothering your food with butter or mystery oil when they cook it.

unsaturated and monounsaturated varieties. Keep saturated fats to a minimum, no more than 10% to 15% of your total calories, and avoid trans fats altogether.

My goal is to weigh what my

driver's license says I weigh. Unknown

Trans fats are right up there in the MADS Hall of Shame with high fructose corn sweetener. Trans fats are made by adding hydrogen to vegetable oil – that's why sometimes they are called hydrogenated (or partially hydrogenated) fats. Food makers love trans fats as ingredients because they have a longer shelf life than regular fats. Unfortunately for people who eat them, trans fats act very much in the same way as saturated fats to clog arteries and raise bad cholesterol levels.

Two other foods to

watch out for

There are a couple of other foods that are "diet killers." There is nothing inherently wrong with these foods, other than they tend to have lots more calories than people think they do.

One of the biggest diet-busters is the bagel. The biggest trap with bagels is portion size. If you look at the nutrition label on most bagel packages, you'll find that about 200 to 300 calories is commonly listed per bagel. The problem is that most bagels sold today are overgrown, humongous descendents of original old-fashioned bagels. So instead of 300 calories or so, your monster-sized bagel you pick up on the way to work may be 600 calories or more. Add some cream cheese or butter and you're having yourself quite a snack there, tubby.

The other innocent looking diet-killer is the muffin. I think I actually hear a reader protesting, "But it's a BRAN muffin!!" Sorry, ace. Like bagels, most muffins have grown into nutritional monstrosities that contain not only mucho calories but in many cases a whole lot of fat. If you're into muffins, look for another way to satisfy the urge – simply look at the nutritional label if you need some incentive to pass up that next muffin.

Thou shalt not weigh more than

thy refrigerator. Anonymous

Chapter Eleven

Our MADS diet strategy

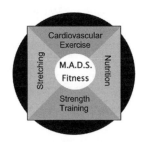

I f you bought this book because you want to lose a few pounds, it's time to listen up. You are about to visit the MADS nutrition boot camp, headed by friendly Sergeant Jim.

Attention recruits! Form two lines! If you want to lose weight fast and get results quickly, get into line A. If you want to lose weight very gradually without as many earth-shattering changes to your diet, choose line B.

Welcome to the MADS Fast Track

If you want to lose weight fast, you can't molly-coddle yourself. We're going to put you on the fast track to great results, but it won't be easy. MADS Fast Track starts with a bang and sets you on a course to lose 10 pounds or more per month.

WEEK ONE

The purpose of this week is to shock your system, establish strict rules that we'll gradually loosen over the following weeks, and get you accustomed to the new foods you'll be enjoying from this point forward. This will be the toughest week, but get through it and you'll not only get fast results but build the foundation for future weight loss.

The rules for WEEK ONE are simple. Remember our A-list foods? Eat as much as you want of the following items from that list. Here are some specific foods to focus on during WEEK ONE:

- **Carrots:** They are an excellent food that's full of vitamins and the crunch gives you a lot of satisfaction. Keep a bag of baby carrots at the ready for snacks.

- **Beans:** Stay away from canned pork and beans, but eat kidney beans, black beans, pinto beans and the like. Beans are an excellent source of protein and fiber. One of my favorite meals when I'm in weight-loss mode is beans with rice and diced chicken breast, mixed with chopped tomatoes (canned or fresh). Season the mixture however you'd like or visit www. MADSfitness.com for recipe ideas.

- **Vegetables and fruits:** Eat all you want of pretty much any vegetable or fresh fruit. The only fruits and veggies that are off limits are corn, peas and avocados. If you cook vegetables, steam them in the microwave or a steamer and if you need fat on them, use a pump spray butter-replacement product (two pumps maximum!). Feel free to season vegetables to your heart's delight except for salt, which you should use sparingly if at all.

- **Salads:** Combine some wonderful A-list veggies into a salad and top it off with low calorie/low fat salad dressing. (Some good ones are Kraft Free® products or Newman's Own® Balsamic Vinaigrette).

- **Soup:** Low in calories and full of veggies, soup is great, if you stay away from cheesy or cream soups and go easy on the crackers.

- **Fish and poultry:** For week one, stick with fish, chicken and turkey instead of beef and pork, and keep careful tabs on portions. Keep a limit of one serving per day of five ounces. A guideline is that a five-ounce portion is about as big as the palm of your hand.

- **Coffee, tea and diet soft drinks:** Although most are on our C-list, these are acceptable "crutches" to get you through the rough moments of the first and following weeks, within limits. A good strategy is to have two diet soft drinks interspersed through the day at the times when you really need something. Bottled green, brown or white tea (artificially sweetened) is a good alternative to diet carbonated sodas, but if we're using this as a crutch it's best to drink the beverages you enjoy. Having a little enjoyment will help you stick to your weight loss plan.

- **Quality protein bars:** These are convenient and can be carried with you. They also have a fair amount of protein (as opposed to cereal bars which have little protein – they are not the same thing!). I prefer Clif® bars and Zone® bars, but there are other good ones on the market. Buy them in multi-pack boxes to keep from going broke. Always check the protein content on the label; 10 grams or more is pretty good, but the higher the better.

- **Water:** During all weeks, drink five or six cups (a cup is eight ounces) of water each and every day. This will help your tummy feel full and will give you something to do to keep you occupied several times a day (if you get my drift).

- **Protein shakes:** If you're doing strength training and eating less red meat than you used to, it's much harder to take in the amount of protein that your body craves. That leads to getting very hungry and possibly falling off the MADS nutrition wagon. That's why I suggest one meal or snack in the form of a protein shake. You can buy protein shake powder in the health section at hipper grocery stores, or go to your local nutrition store. If that doesn't work for you, surf to www.bodybuilding.com and have it shipped to you. There are different kinds of protein powder, but I suggest whey protein. Don't go for the more sophisticated stuff with all the fancy scientific reasons why it costs more; stick with basic whey protein. Expect to pay about $25 to $30 for a big canister of powder (compared to meat, that's a lot of protein for your hard-earned dollar). You'll be living with the canister for well over a month, so I suggest vanilla flavor because it mixes with other ingredients better. Although you can mix whey powder with milk or water and drink it, a more enjoyable way is to mix it in a blender with a little milk or soy milk, some water, one-half banana (or other fruit) and a handful of ice.

Not allowed in WEEK ONE:

- Except for the exceptions just mentioned, anything not on the A-list

- Sugar (artificial sweeteners are OK)

- Beef, pork or other red meats

- Alcohol of any kind (it slows your body's fat burning)

- Bread, rolls, crackers, donuts, muffins and similar items

Smaller portions but more often

There's a diet trick that can work very well – or it can backfire miserably. It is important to do it properly and pay attention to portion control. Instead of eating three or maybe four times a day, eat five or six times each day. This takes a bit more planning because you obviously are not eating full meals on all six occasions.

Here is a daily schedule that has worked for me, but you can set up your own schedule that best serves you:

❗ MADS Tip!

6 a.m.	Breakfast (oatmeal with fruit and milk)
9 a.m.	Protein shake or bar (200 calories or so)
Noon	Fruit or leftover rice and beans (200 calories or so)
3 p.m.	Fruit or protein bar (200 calories or so)
6 p.m.	Dinner (one portion of meat, brown rice or baked potato and salad)
9 p.m.	Glass of fat-free milk or fruit

How this helps is that you always have something to eat on the horizon so you don't feel like you are depriving yourself. The pitfall is that you can end up chowing down a regular-sized portion six times a day instead of three. That's a disaster if you're trying to lose weight. The idea is to eat more often but take in fewer calories per session.

What to expect in WEEK ONE

I'm not going to blow sunshine up your skirt – WEEK ONE is no picnic. But stick with it! If you follow the rules for WEEK ONE you'll get outstanding results. Chances are you'll lose some impressive poundage in WEEK ONE, because there is a lot of water sloshing around inside you that's trapped in bloated fat cells. Interestingly, when you gain weight you don't add more fat cells – the fat cells you have just get bigger and bigger. When your fat cells shrink they will give up water. So your weight loss in WEEK ONE will reflect not only actual fat loss, but considerable water as well. I have lost up to 12 pounds during a WEEK ONE regimen.

I eat whatever the guy who

beat me in the

last race ate. Alex Ratelle

Try not to avoid becoming obsessed with weighing yourself. Your weight fluctuates in the short term so you'll only become discouraged if you check your weight too often. If you can pull it off, try to avoid the scale completely for seven full days. If you can't resist stepping on the scale, do it every other day at the most.

As WEEK ONE wears on, you should become less hungry but you will still have plenty of times when you crave naughty foods. That's natural – you're not going to overcome many years of eating habits in just a few days.

Exercising during WEEK ONE

I'm going to leave it up to you how much (or even if) you exercise in WEEK ONE. Focus on sticking closely to the nutrition plan – that is more important than exercise during the first week. If you are accustomed to exercising and it's already part of your day-to-day routine, by all means you should continue with your current exercise program. But WEEK ONE is not the time to start a brand new exercise program, especially one that is aggressive.

If you are not exercising right now, you should use WEEK ONE to get your motor going a bit without overdoing it. Take a leisurely walk each day and start performing the basic stretching routine, appropriately found in the section of this book entitled "Stretching."

WEEK TWO AND THREE:

If you stuck to your guns during WEEK ONE you have lost some weight but are ready for a little more variety and fun in your diet.

During WEEK TWO AND THREE have all of the foods permitted in WEEK ONE plus...

- **Nuts:** These are great sources of protein and good fats, but they are very calorie dense. Pay close attention to portion size when eating nuts. Use a small measuring cup to dole out a single serving – don't eat nuts right out of the can! Peanut butter is also OK, but we aren't allowed to eat bread, rolls or crackers yet so eating peanut butter by itself can be a sticky situation.

- **Yogurt:** This is another calorie-dense food with many positives including protein. Choose the low fat and sugar-free varieties, and stay away from the "fruit on the bottom" style.

- **White potatoes:** Spuds are a much-maligned food but the fault lies mostly in what we do with potatoes, such as French fries and drenching them with butter and sour cream. We're only going to eat them baked, and use seasonings and a couple of hits of pump-style margarine to add flavor.

- **Breakfast cereals:** Not sugar-laden cereals, which are bad. The best choices for cereals are the plain old stand-bys like corn flakes, shredded wheat, Grape Nuts® brand and similar cereals. Cereal can be a good choice for one of your lighter "meals," but watch your portions.

- **Lean beef and lean pork:** We are still keeping to five ounces of fish or meat per day, but now you can add beef and pork to your options.

- **Eggs:** Preferably have your eggs boiled or poached to hold the fat down, but scrambled or fried using only cooking spray for preparation is OK. Eggs have gotten a bad rap in the past, mostly because of the various high-fat ways of preparing them. Up to four eggs a week can be a good source of protein. Egg whites or egg substitute products (like Egg Beaters® brand) are an even better choice than whole eggs, but if you prefer whole eggs then go for it.

Rules for success in WEEKS TWO AND THREE:

During WEEK ONE you learned the basic habits, and we'll continue to reinforce those during the next two weeks. Remember:

- Small portions

- Eat five to six times a day

- Keep drinking six 8-ounce glasses of water each day

- Be vigilant with portion control – measure everything except for

fruits and vegetables

Exercising during WEEKS TWO AND THREE:

Now that your body has had a week of getting fewer calories, your metabolism will start to slow down. Your body thinks there's a full-fledged famine going on

The biggest challenges in WEEKS TWO AND THREE for most people **MADS Tip!** are: (1) maintaining portion control, (2) being tempted by some of the foods you crave and (3) not seeing weight loss results as fast as you'd like. To head these challenges off at the pass, be extra careful about portions and keep telling yourself that this is only two weeks out of your long lifetime. The sacrifices you are making in WEEK TWO AND THREE won't kill you – but the effects of bad eating habits could!

and will try to cut metabolism before using the fat it has stored away. Good news if there were really a famine, bad news if you're trying to shed pounds.

But we have a trick up our sleeves to fool good old Mother Nature, and that's exercise. WEEK TWO is the time when we're going to exercise and kick our metabolism into a higher gear. That will push your body to a new level of fat burning and overcome its tendency to slow down your metabolism.

Dieting is wishful

shrinking! Anonymous

Gradually work into an exercise routine. Set up a routine of three to four days a week of exercise with stretching on your "rest" days. Don't over-do the intensity of exercise – read and heed the cautions in the CV and strength training chapters about starting with minimal weight and a somewhat leisurely pace.

Here is an example of a good routine for WEEKS TWO AND THREE:

Sunday	Cardio exercise + stretching
Monday	Strength training + stretching
Tuesday	Cardio exercise + stretching
Wednesday	Stretching
Thursday	Strength training + stretching
Friday	Cardio exercise + stretching
Saturday	Stretching

WEEK FOUR:

If you've stuck with it so far, you've laid a fantastic foundation for future eating habits and you've probably lost anywhere from 6 to 15 pounds. If you're closer to or less than the lower number, don't be discouraged – how many pounds you lose depends on what your starting weight was and a lot of other factors.

We're going to loosen the rules up a bit here in WEEK FOUR. You can have all of the items permitted during the past three weeks, plus add the following:

- A slice of bread or one small roll per day
- An extra 5 ounces of meat *per week*, besides the 5 ounces per day you're already allowed
- Beer or wine, up to two servings (a serving is 12 ounces beer or 6 ounces wine) *per week*
- For meat choice, add LEAN cold cuts (turkey, chicken, etc.)

If that doesn't spell P-A-R-T-Y then I don't know what does!

The trap of reduced calorie foods

It seems these days like every food has a "light" or low calorie or low fat or sugar free version. It doesn't matter how inherently unhealthy a food may be, you can buy a version that is supposed to be OK when you're dieting. Sorry to break your bubble, but the MADS program doesn't allow these. Ice cream, donuts, cookies and their fattening cousins are considered D-list or F-list foods for your MADS nutrition program, no matter what promises the label makes.

People worry about what they eat

between Christmas and the New Year's Day, but they

really should worry about what they eat

between the New Year's Day and Christmas. Unknown

One of the goals of the MADS nutrition program is to get you to learn to like naturally healthy foods like vegetables and fruits. Hopefully, you'll pick up some good habits that will stick with you in the long run. You may get short term results from substituting low calorie foods for their high calorie counterparts, but in the long haul you'll slip back into your old habits and those lost pounds will find their way back to your backside as if they were using a tiny little global positioning system to hunt you down.

Studies have shown that, when people eat "light" versions of high calorie foods, there is a tendency is to simply eat more of the "light" food so that they end up with the same amount (or more) calories. That being the case, the only weight you'll end up losing is in your wallet because you've taken a double hit to your food budget: you paid a premium price for the "light" version and you've eaten two times more of it.

Dealing with a bad day

Even self-proclaimed fitness gods that are soon-to-be best-selling authors have bad eating days. Special occasions or just a lapse of willpower can cause a detour from your goals.

A common result of having a slip-up is guilt. You find yourself thinking, "I've worked so hard and now (like the last ten times I've tried to lose weight) I've failed," and then proceed to drown your sorrows in a box of cookies. The result can be what I call the REALLY BAD DAY. The thought process goes, "Today is a bust anyway so I may as well cut loose and eat everything that isn't nailed down."

With the MADS program, we forgive a bad day now and then – as long as the bad days don't start coming one after another. Our rules about bad days are:

- Don't make a bad day worse by giving up for the entire day. Think about it this way: If you slip up and eat 1,000 calories too many, you haven't done so much damage that you can't make it up over the next few days. But if you keep going and overeat by 5,000 calories, you've not only ruined your day but pretty much the whole week. So keep your slip-ups isolated.

- Live by the rule, "Once is a slip-up, twice is a habit." If you have a bad day, set your mind to having a good following day. When it comes to slip-ups, we'll declare a "cheat day," where you can slip up once in awhile but make up for it on the other days.

Avoid falling into the "incremental trap"

When you're trying to lose weight, you walk a fine line between eating enough to maintain enough energy to function, and not eating too much where you won't lose weight. Your own body is your worst enemy in trying to stay on that fine line, because it will sabotage your conscious weight loss efforts. We can live with the obvious hunger pangs, but as your nutrition program extends over days and weeks, you can easily fall into what I call the "incremental trap." That's where you add just a little bit onto how much you eat, or maybe choose foods that aren't too bad, but not as good as the ones you chose a few weeks earlier in your nutrition program. Pretty soon your weight loss levels off and you hit a plateau.

Let's look at an example of how this can happen. Say you eat a small bowl of cereal with milk as your 9 p.m. snack. During your first week or two you carefully measure one serving of cereal and milk, but as time goes on you start to guesstimate the amount you put in your bowl instead of measuring it. Your cereal portion creeps up a little bit, maybe just a few pieces each day, until you have increased your serving size by 20% or more in just a couple of weeks.

That's one example of the "incremental trap," which can rear its ugly head in many ways. Now that you're aware of it, be continually vigilant so that it doesn't happen to you.

Practice the lost art of portion control

If you ask foreign visitors to describe American eating habits, many mention how large American portions are compared to other parts of the world. Over the last couple of decades, we have somehow gotten accustomed to portion sizes that are a lot bigger than they were in the past.

Portion control is nothing more than a learning process. You'll have to pay close attention to it for awhile until your eye gets used to smaller portion sizes.

But we're not going to go overboard on this – if you don't already own a portion scale, don't run out and buy one. A measuring cup comes in handy, however.

When it comes to meat or fish, we'll use the good old "deck of cards" or "palm of hand" guidelines which say a 5-ounce portion is about the size of a deck of cards or your palm. For most other items, we'll count on our trusty measuring cup. Simply refer to the product label for serving size and measure out that amount.

Fruits and veggies are great because, even in cases where you need to guess portion size, it's difficult to eat a large enough amount of fruit or vegetables to do any damage to your weight loss goals. That's why we include most fruits and veggies on our A-list – they are foolproof foods for weight loss success.

If you're eating packaged foods, which we try to keep to a minimum, pay special attention to portion sizes. A small bag of mixed nuts, for example, may look like a single serving but contain two or three servings. You can easily end up tripling the number of calories you thought you were eating. Read the nutritional label before you open the bag or box, and limit yourself to one serving.

WEEK X: Adapting for the long haul

By now, you have probably lost from 10 pounds to 20 pounds. If you're not at your goal weight yet, here are your options:

- If you're making progress that you're happy with, stick to the WEEK 4 rules indefinitely until you reach your goal weight.
- If you've wandered off the straight and narrow path and haven't got-

ten anywhere near the results you wanted, try repeating WEEK ONE and WEEK TWO again. This will hopefully get you back on track and give you a quick jump-start in terms of results. After completing WEEK TWO, come back to WEEK FOUR.

• If you've made progress but aren't particularly happy with your results, jump back to WEEK TWO for a week, then return to WEEK FOUR.

Stay on the X-PLAN until you reach your goal weight and, (to steal from Gene Hackman in "Hoosiers") "You *will* reach your goal weight," then use the X-PLAN to help you maintain that weight. The X-PLAN simply stated is:

Follow WEEK FOUR rules for at least 5 days each week, preferably 6 days (I usually follow the rules Monday through Friday) and on the other two days, allow yourself to have one or two things you wouldn't normally have. But keep this within reason – if you want a donut, have one donut, not two or three. Remember, these are off days, not "anything goes" days. By now after several weeks of health eating, your body has learned to send you signals if you're over-indulging. Listen to your body's signals and you'll maintain your weight. Gradually return to ignoring these warnings and you'll put back the weight in no time.

Also very important in the X-PLAN is your exercise program. If you've embraced (OK, maybe not embraced but you grudgingly went along with it) strength training, cardiovascular exercise and stretching, you have the key to keeping that weight off in the long haul.

Is there anyone still in the gradual weight loss line?

Did you pick line B, the gradual weight loss line, at the start of this chapter? Do you remember the start of this chapter? If you are looking for gradual weight loss, your directions are pretty straightforward:

(1) Start your weight loss plan at WEEK FOUR as described earlier and follow the WEEK FOUR plan for as long as you need to in order to lose the desired weight. At a minimum, stick with it for at least three weeks, as it may take some time to see noticeable results.

(2) Follow the MADS program of strength training, cardiovascular exercise and stretching starting right away in your first week.

(3) If you get stuck on the way, try following the WEEK ONE plan for at least four or five days – that should get you back on track.

Assuming you are following all four parts of the MADS program, you should burn an extra 1,500 calories or more per week exercising as well as take in fewer calories than you were before. That should result in at least a one to two pound weight loss per week.

How calories work and how much food is too much

Remember when we said food is like fuel for our bodies? A calorie is actually a measure of energy, so a food with lots of calories has more energy in it than a lower calorie food. If you don't use the excess energy, roughly 1,400 calories go into a pound of fat.

There are two ways to lose weight: increase the rate at which you burn calories and/or take in fewer calories. In MADS, the combination of eating lower calorie foods and exercising aggressively is what provides supercharged, long term weight loss results.

What can we learn from the information in the box shown below? First, old Father Time is out to screw us every step of the way by slowing our metabolism as we get older. Second, the more active a person is the more calories they use. Chances are that you would be considered sedentary or mildly active right now. The MADS exercise program will put you squarely in the "very active" category,

MADS Tip!

The number of calories a person requires each day depends on age (a real bummer for us middle-aged folks), activity level, current size and sex (not whether you have sex or not, but on your gender). Here are some examples of calories used per day.

Calories burned per day

	Male Person		Female Person	
	Age 40	Age 50	Age 40	Age 50
Sedentary	2,080	2,020	1,640	1,580
Mildly Active	2,383	2,314	1,880	1,811
Very Active	2,989	2,903	2,358	2,272

which means you'll be burning at least 400 calories more per day (and maybe up to 900 calories daily, depnding on your current activity level) than you are now. The difference in number of calories used in varying activity levels may not seem like a lot, but assuming all else stays the same and you burn an extra 400 calories per day through exercise, you could end up losing two pounds or more per week just from the change in your metabolism.

MADS Tip!

Everything we talked about so far can be wrapped up in this simple equation:

Better food choices + MADS exercise program

= you become a lean, mean, calorie burning machine

Chapter Twelve

Stretching

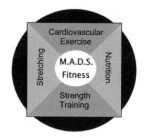

We've spent a lot of time talking about strength training, cardiovascular exercise and nutrition. But remember: our fitness chair has four legs, not three. You might be able to sit in a three-legged chair but it wouldn't be very sturdy. As the fourth leg of our fitness chair, stretching isn't an absolute necessity – but it gives you some important fitness bennies that the other three parts of the MADS program don't.

Stretching: A good investment of a few minutes a day

The biggest reason to spend a few minutes a day stretching is to increase your flexibility. As we get older, muscles are more likely to tighten up, and strength training can make the situation worse because it tends to tighten muscles. If you do regular stretching, chances are that you'll find it easier to bend, twist and do all the other movements that are required in daily life.

Another way stretching helps is to increase blood flow into the area being stretched, and this blood flow helps heal and rejuvenate muscles, ligaments and tendons. A lot of aches and pains that you might experience on a day-to-day basis can be improved, even eliminated, by including stretching in your overall fitness routine. Stop complaining about your aches and pains and start stretching!

I'll admit that I have not always been a big fan of stretching. In the past I looked at it as the weak sister (or sibling, if you prefer the gender non-specific term) in my fitness routine. If I was short on time, stretching is what I would jettison – I'd sometimes skip it even if I wasn't in a hurry. Then I suffered a pesky strain in my lower calf and Achilles tendon that lingered on and on for months. I tried everything – a trip to the doctor, heat pads, ice packs, rest, aspirin, you name it. Nothing helped until I started spending just a couple of minutes a day stretching my calves and Achilles tendons. That did the trick, and I've been a big fan of stretching ever since.

Few people realize it, but tight muscles can result in pain in other parts of the body. Tight calves, for instance, can cause the *plantar fascia* (a thin sheet-like tendon that stretches from your heel to the front of your foot near the base of your toes) to stretch so tight that it develops tiny tears. If you've never experienced this, you get a cookie. But if you've had this condition, you know how uncomfortable it is. Calf stretches are a great way to prevent and even help alleviate this painful condition if you've already got it.

We've seen there are lots of reasons why you should stretch. If you're convinced, you might be wondering: when should I do stretching? Any time that you can fit it in and any place! Unlike strength training and cardio, stretching doesn't require any special equipment and only takes five or ten minutes. The beauty of stretching is that you can do it any time of the day, just about anywhere you'd like.

Gyms usually have areas with mats that are set aside for stretching, but a carpeted floor at home works just as well. Your office floor (assuming it has been vacuumed at least once in the new millennium) works fine too, if you have 10 minutes to spare while the boss isn't around.

A basic stretching routine

First, we're going to lay out a set of basic stretching exercises that can be done in just 5 or 10 minutes. Then we'll wrap up the stretching discussion with a few simple guidelines to remember.

Start the basic stretching routine by lying flat on your back.

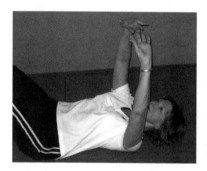

Stretch #1 – Shoulders: Extend your arms straight above your face. Now turn your palms up to the ceiling with your fingers pointing toward each other. Interlock your fingers and, keeping your arms straight, slowly bring your arms above your head while keeping your fingers interlocked and elbows as straight as possible. Hold for this position for 30 seconds and slowly return to the starting position. Release your hands and get ready for the next stretch – we haven't got all day, you know.

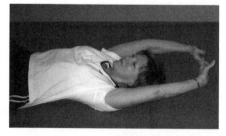

Stretch #2 – Hips: Still lying on your back, slowly raise your right leg and bend the knee, bringing the knee up toward your chest. Grab your upper thigh with both

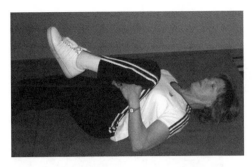

hands to help. Hold for 30 seconds, then release and repeat with your left leg.

Stretch #3 – Groin area: Sit up and bend your legs so that the soles of your feet are against one another. Use your hands to slowly press your knees toward the floor, although you probably won't be able to get them to actually touch the floor. Hold for 30 seconds and release.

Stretch #4 – Double H - Hips n' Hamstrings: While sitting on the mat or floor, extend your left leg straight, while bending your right leg into the position shown. The edge of your right foot should be touching your left thigh and your left leg should have

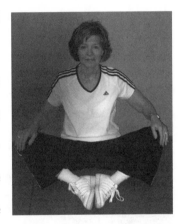

the knee straight or bent just a tiny bit. Enjoy the right hip stretch for about 20 seconds. Now slowly bend forward at the waist. You'll start to feel a stretch behind the knee and into your upper leg pretty quickly. When you feel the stretch, hold that position for about 20 seconds. Release and do the same thing with the other leg.

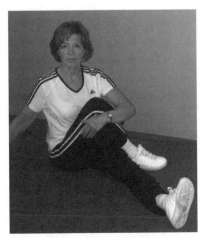

Stretch #5 – Back extensions: Now lie

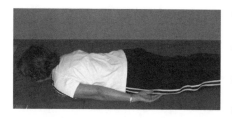

on your stomach with hands at your sides and legs out straight. Lift up your head up as high as you can while looking straight ahead and arch your back. Let your feet

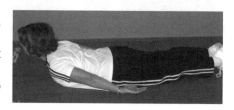

come off the floor a little bit if you want to. Hold a second or two, and release. Repeat this movement 10 times to start and try to work up to 20 or more.

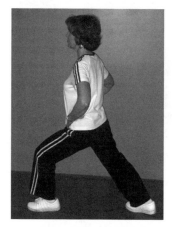

Stretch #6 – Calves: Start in a standing position with your feet together. Depending on how good your balance is, it may help to be near a wall or chair you can use to rest your hand on to keep your balance. Now step forward with your left foot and back with

your right. Try to keep your right heel on the floor and lean slightly

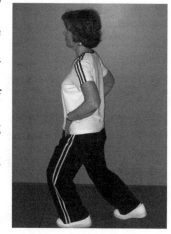

forward. You should feel a stretch in your right calf area. Hold this position for 20-30 seconds. Now bring your right foot forward a bit and, while still keeping your heel on the floor, try to drop your right knee toward the floor. You won't get far with it and you will

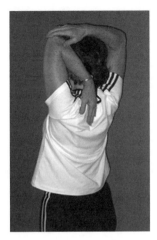

feel a stretch in your Achilles tendon area near your heel. Now do the same two movements with the other leg.

Stretch #7 – Back scratchers: How often do you have an itch that you just can't scratch? Those days are over after you do this stretch for a couple of weeks. Stand up, and with your left arm reach back over your shoulder and try to scratch the middle of your back. Try to keep your shoulder in normal position. If it helps, use your other hand to pull lightly on your elbow as shown in the photo. Reach as far as you can, hold for 30 seconds and repeat with the other arm.

The routine we just laid out covers the basics, but visit www.MADSfitness.com for some body-part-specific stretching routines if you have some trouble spots you'd like to focus on. Here is an important point: If you have a health problem with any of the body parts you are stretching, get your doctor's OK before doing that particular stretch, or just skip that stretch.

Once you get the hang of the little routine we are using, you should be able to git'r done in under 10 minutes. There's no need to rest in between stretches; in fact the routine we just talked about is set up to transition efficiently between one stretch and the next with no stopping.

If you feel ambitious and like stretching, work up to 2 or 3 stretching intervals of 30 seconds each for each stretch. Shoot for 30 seconds, but no longer than that.

Your personal fitness guru agrees with the other self-proclaimed experts who say that there isn't any big benefit from holding stretches longer than 30 seconds.

Make sure that you feel your muscles stretch – if you don't feel a noticeable pull in the area you are stretching, you're either doing the motion incorrectly or not stretching as far as you could. After doing this stretching routine for just a few days, you should start to notice at least a little improved flexibility. Keep pushing your limits and your flexibility will continue to improve, in many cases dramatically, over weeks and months.

One of the big rules of stretching is that you should never bounce. Bouncing can pull or tear muscles. Stretching should always be a smooth and slow movement. Inch yourself little by little into the full stretch position, and once you are in that stretch position simply hold it, but don't bounce.

If you only remember a hundred things from this book, make this one of them: In stretching, you get out of it what you put into it. Don't just go through the motions, but try to stretch a little further every time. If you're doing it right, you will be rewarded with a definite improvement in range-of-motion and overall flexibility within a couple of weeks of stretching.

Unlike strength training where you absolutely should have a rest day in between workouts, you can feel free to stretch every day if you'd like. Sometimes the best way to make sure you don't skip your stretching is to make it either a part of your daily routine or part of your standard workout. One idea is to do your stretching every time you do your cardio exercise. In any event, make sure you stretch at least every other day.

That's it! If everything in life were as simple as stretching, the world would be a better place, would it not?

Chapter Thirteen

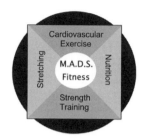

Put it all together and it spells MADS

All right, you've stuck with me this long so let's wrap this baby up and tie it with a nice red bow.

We said at the beginning that MADS is a four-part program that will get you in the best shape that you've been in for a long, long time. To make MADS work effectively, you need to participate in all four parts: (1) strength training, (2) cardiovascular exercise, (3) stretching and (4) proper nutrition.

Like I said a number of times, the important thing is that you get started. At this moment, you are just 60 days away from looking and feeling years younger. All you have to do is pull the trigger and get going! When you put down this book in a minute or two, pick up a pad of paper and start working on your plan. Make a grocery list with lots of A-list and B-list foods and few if any D-list and F-list foods. Decide if you'll exercise at home or at a health club. If you choose the health club route, look up the phone numbers for a couple of health clubs in your area and make an appointment for a tour. Lay out a realistic schedule for when you will do strength training, stretching and cardio. *Then do it!*

I stressed before that if you can't carry out MADS to perfection, then shoot for 90%. If you can't do 90%, then strive for 80%. If 80% isn't possible, then try for 70%. The important thing is to *start now* and take positive steps – you can aim for perfection later.

Well, it's time for me to punch out. The only question that remains is: When I win the Nobel Prize for Literature, do they pay the prize money out all at once or in payments like they do if you win the lottery?

Seriously, thanks to you for reading this book and placing your trust in me to help you with your health and fitness. Hopefully you had a few laughs (OK, maybe a chuckle or two) in reading this book, but believe me when I say that your fitness and well-being is something I take very seriously.

Get started and also try to have fun while you're doing it. My best wishes are with you in reaching your fitness goals. Be sure to email me at jlaabs@firstamericanpublishing.com and let me know how you're doing.

Appendix

Strength Training Exercises

Quad lifts (a.k.a. leg curls)

Comments: Generally requires either a machine or a bench with an attachment

Primary muscles affected: Quadriceps

Narrative: Adjust the pad so you are pushing with your upper ankle area. Bring your legs up slowly until they are straight. Then slowly lower the weight back down.

Sets and reps: Work up to three sets of 8 to 10 reps each.

Weight level: This is generally a high weight exercise, and you should see rapid improvement in the amount of weight that you use.

Checkpoints: Make sure to adjust the seatback so your knee joints line up with the pivot point of the machine. Keep your butt touching the seat. Use a full range of motion as shown below.

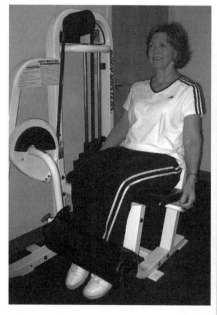

Start

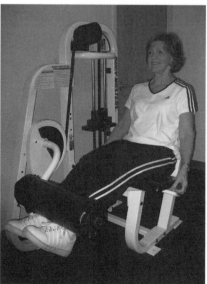

Midpoint

Hamstring curls

Comments: Requires a machine or bench with attachment. There are two machine types – in one you lay on your belly, the other is from a seated position. Some home machines require you to stand on one leg and work the other leg.

Muscles affected: Hamstrings, secondarily the gluteus (a nice way of saying the rear end).

Narrative: Locate foot pad so that it contacts your lower calf area just above the ankle. Bend your knees until your feet are as close to your rear as is comfortable, then slowly allow weight to return to starting position.

Sets and reps: Work up to three sets of 8-10 reps each.

Weight level: Try to maintain a ratio of at least two-thirds of the weight you use for quad lifts. (If you are using 120 pounds for quad lifts, use 80 pounds for hamstring curls.)

Checkpoints: Make sure to adjust the machine so your knee joints line up with the pivot point of the machine. Be sure to use a full range of motion.

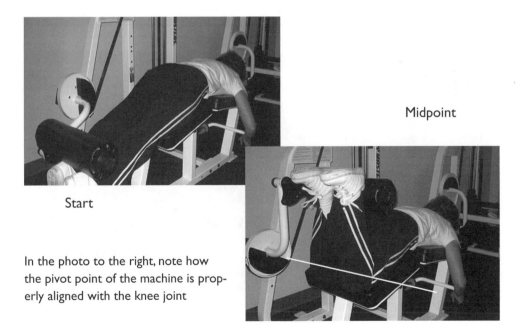

Midpoint

Start

In the photo to the right, note how the pivot point of the machine is properly aligned with the knee joint

Bench press

Comments: This exercise is a part of just about any self-respecting strength training program, including MADS, so pay attention. Machines tend to be safer and more effective because you can use higher weights without needing a spotter.

Muscles affected: Primarily the chest with secondary involvement from the deltoids (shoulders) and triceps.

Sets and reps: Work up to three sets of 10 reps each.

Weight level: This is a mid-to-high weight exercise, but start with relatively low weights until you get the hang of it. That's especially important if you are using free weights as your torso and face will be the first stopping point for any weights that you drop.

Checkpoints: Your hands should be at or slightly above/below the nipple line. Try not to arch your back as you push the weight; instead try to keep your hips and lower back against the bench or the back pad. Don't forget proper breathing.

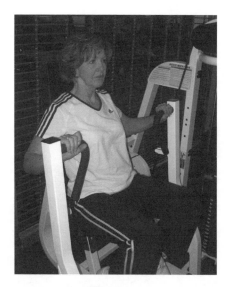

Start

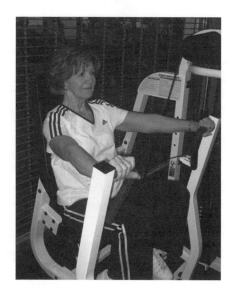

Midpoint

Calf raises
(not pictured)

Comments: Can be done on a variety of machines, with free weights or with no weights on a step in your home. You can do this exercise with no weights and get benefits.

Muscles affected: Calf muscles.

Narrative: Starting with your calves stretched (heels down), you push up your feet until you are standing on your tip toes, pause a moment and then return to starting position.

Sets and reps: Work up to three sets of 12-15 reps each.

Weight level: Generally this is a heavier weight exercise, but if you have back, knee, hip, or shoulder problems choose a machine where you do the exercise in a seated position If you have foot, ankle or Achilles tendon problems, avoid this exercise.

Checkpoints: Be sure to pause both at the bottom and top of the motion. Also go through the full motion, by stretching your heel down as far as is comfortable and pushing up as far as possible.

Bend-overs
(not pictured)

Comments: Have you ever heard the one about the two male prisoners in the shower? One approaches the other and says, "Bend over!" to which the other replies, "Glad to meet you, Ben." This exercise can be done with a barbell, with no weight at all, or it can be done on a specialized piece of gym equipment.

Muscles affected: Lower back, with some hamstring and hip involvement

Sets and reps: Work up to three sets of 10 reps each.

Weight level: This is a middle weight exercise, but start with low weights. This is an exercise to avoid if you have lower back problems. It is not in our basic routine.

Checkpoints: If you're doing this with a barbell, stick your butt out a little. Also, only bend as far as you feel comfortable with. Try low weights or no weights to get the feel of it and stretch your back muscles.

Rows

Comments: Can be done on a variety of machines or with free weights.

Muscles affected: Middle and upper back, but involves much of the upper body including shoulders and arms.

Sets and reps: Work up to three sets of 10 reps each.

Narrative: Slowly pull the weight back (or up) toward you, while keeping your elbows close to your body and trying to pinch your shoulder blades together.

Weight level: This is a mid-to-heavy weight exercise, but start with low weights and work up to heavier weights, especially if you have back or shoulder problems.

Checkpoints: When you pull the weight toward you, your hands should the height of the lower chest area. Avoid these two common "cheats": (1) In the negative portion, be sure to let your arms become almost straight; not just part of the way, and (2) Don't lean backwards when pulling the handle toward you; try to remain seated straight.

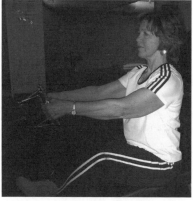
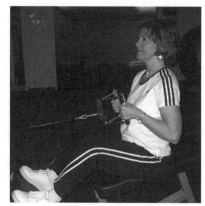

Start   Midpoint

Lat pull-downs

Comments: Can be done on a variety of machines; if you have no machines available to you, this exercise is basically a pull up (sometimes called a chin up).

Muscles affected: Upper back, but involves shoulders and arms.

Sets and reps: Work up to three sets of 10 reps each.

Weight level: This is a mid-to-heavy weight exercise, but start with low weights and work up to heavier weights, especially if you have shoulder problems.

Checkpoints: Be sure to pull the weight to the front about to collarbone level (not lower), and *not* behind your head. The biggest "cheat" on this exercise is leaning back while you pull down, which turns the exercise into a row and works your mid-back instead of your upper back.

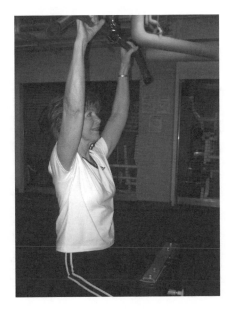

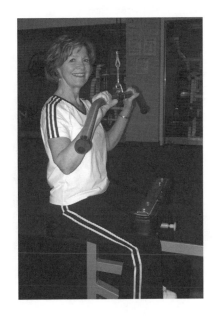

Start   Midpoint

Chest flyes

Comments: Another classic movement and staple of the exercise world. It is demonstrated here with dumbbells but there are also machines that allow you to do this exercise.

Muscles affected: Chest area

Sets and reps: Work up to three sets of 10 reps each.

Weight level: Start low because you're working muscles that probably haven't been worked in awhile. Expect some soreness in your chest at first.

Checkpoints: The main way to hurt yourself is by starting with the weights too far back (on a machine) or too low (if laying on your back with dumbbells). Your hands should never be lower than the bench or behind the line of the backrest on a machine. On a machine, I usually use the front-most starting position.

Start

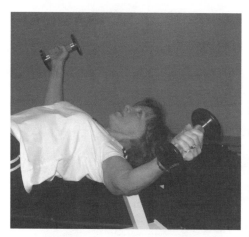

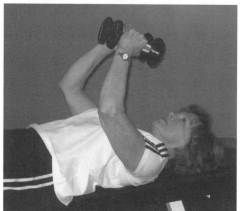

Midpoint

Squats/leg presses

Comments: I suggest either using a machine or doing this exercise with little or no weight as pictured, especially if you're new to strength training. Squatting with low or no extra weight can be beneficial, just use higher reps.

Muscles affected: Thighs and hips, also all leg muscles and lower back.

Narrative: This exercise involves squatting, then returning your legs to an almost straight position.

Sets and reps: Work up to three sets of 10-12 reps each, 15-25 with low or no weight.

Weight level: Generally this is a heavier weight exercise, but if you have back, knee, hip or ankle problems you should either avoid this exercise or use very modest weights.

Checkpoints: Never bend your knees further than a 90-degree angle. Also never lock your knees in the straight leg part of the movement.

Start

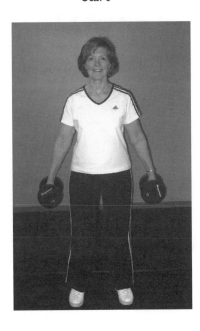

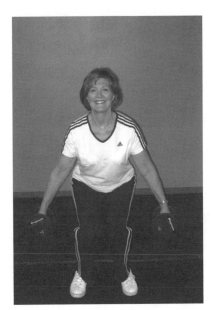

Midpoint

Basic biceps curls

Comments: There are probably more variations to arm curls than any other exercise. This is the plain vanilla version and is pictured using dumbbells although there are a number of machines for curls.

Muscles affected: Biceps with some involvement from the forearms and front portion of your shoulder muscles (deltoids).

Sets and reps: Work up to three sets of 10 reps each.

Weight level: Relative to other exercises, this movement uses fairly low weight.

Checkpoints: Be sure to use the entire range of motion, especially on the downward part of the motion. Stay seated if you're using a machine. Keep hands about shoulder width apart. Watch your pace!

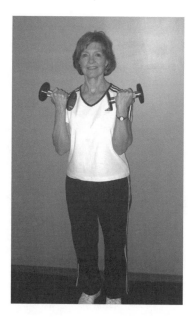

Midpoint

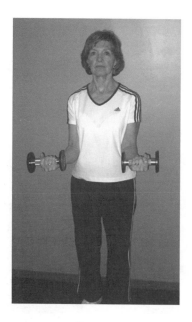

Start

Triceps curls

Comments: This is a good exercise for anyone, but women can benefit a lot because it tightens the muscles in the back part of the upper arm, which is often a trouble spot. It is shown with dumbbells but there are also machines for this exercise

Narrative: Start with the weights in front of your forehead and arms bent. Then push the weights away from you and straighten your arms. Keep your elbows as motionless as possible. Then slowly bring the weight back toward your forehead.

Muscles affected: Triceps muscle area, the back of your upper arms.

Sets and reps: Work up to three sets of 10 reps each.

Weight level: Probably the lowest of any strength training exercise.

Checkpoints: Use the whole range of motion, especially when your hands are coming back toward you. Try not to move your elbows, they should be the pivot joint; also, there is a tendency to let them stick out to the side a bit, so keep them in line with your shoulders. If using free weights, be careful or you'll learn why this exercise is called the "skull crusher."

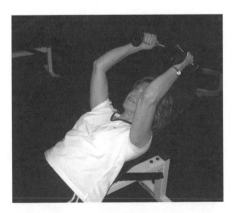

Start

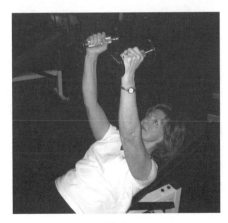

Midpoint

Dips and triceps push downs

Comments: There are various devices on which to perform this exercise but you can do this just as well on an exercise bench (pitured below), chair or coffee table. This is not part of our basic routine but if you are concerned about the backs of your arms being flabby, you can add this exercise onto your list.

Muscles affected: Triceps muscle area, but with an emphasis on a slightly different muscle portion than triceps curls.

Sets and reps: Work up to three sets of 10-15 reps each.

Weight level: On a dip rack or using a bench, your body is the weight. If using a machine this is a middle level weight exercise.

Checkpoints: Never go beyond a 90 degree bend at your elbow to avoid injury. Keep your elbows parallel to your body as much as possible rather than letting them stick out to the sides as is the natural tendency.

Midpoint

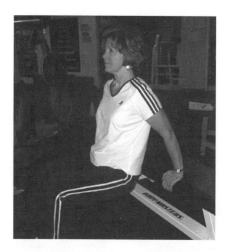

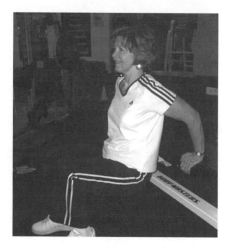

Start

Side raises

Comments: This is a good shoulder exercise that can be done with dumbbells or on a machine.

Muscles affected: Deltoids(shoulders)

Sets and reps: Work up to three sets of 10 reps each.

Weight level: Relatively low weights. If you have shoulder problems try this with very low weights and if you feel any pain, skip this exercise.

Checkpoints: Be sure to pause a bit at the bottom of the motion to avoid using momentum to make the exercise easier. To avoid injury, don't lift the weights higher than shoulder level. If using a machine, the pivot point should he in line with your shoulder joint.

Start

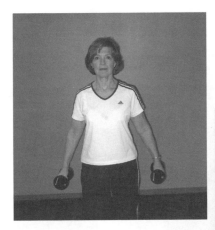

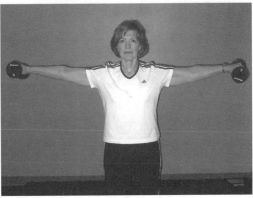

Midpoint

Overhead presses

Comments: A classic exercise and good for the shoulders.

Muscles affected: Deltoids, mostly the front and top peaks but not the rear deltoids.

Sets and reps: Work up to three sets of 10 reps each.

Weight level: Relatively low weights. Be very careful as shoulder injury can occur if you use too much weight or improper form. If you have shoulder problems, start with extremely low weights and if you feel pain, skip this exercise.

Checkpoints: Don't lower the weight to the point where your elbows are beyond 90 degrees. It's best to do this exercise sitting with a lower back support. That not only helps prevent injury but keeps you from cheating by leaning back.

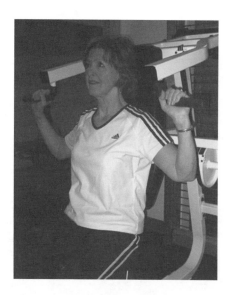

Start

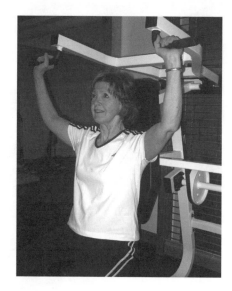

Midpoint

Total ab crunches

Comments: This is the standard version of crunch, with your feet straight out. For variation, try resting your legs on an elevated object like an ottoman. This is one of countless versions of crunch; I like this one because it works most of the general ab area. You can do these anywhere, at home on the floor or on a mat in the gym.

Muscles affected: Some lower ab involvement but this primarily hits the middle area of your tummy from your belly button to your lower ribcage.

Sets and reps: I prefer one set with a lot of repetitions; 50 to 60 reps once you're in the swing of things. Start with at least 20 reps in one set. It takes a certain number of reps just to get these muscles working.

Checkpoints: Don't interlock your fingers behind your head; that can cause a neck injury. Try it as shown without your hands behind your head. As you do the crunch, visualize trying to force your belly button down through the floor. Watch your pace, slower is better.

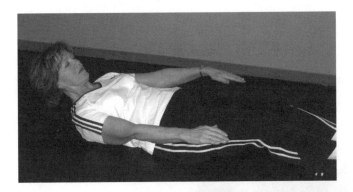

Midpoint

Start

Photo Model:
Sharon Hahn

Thanks to Core Athletic, LLC in
Middleton, Wisconsin for use of
their facility for photos

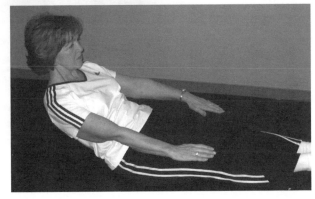

Tighten-ups

Comments: Who says you can't squeeze in some ab work while you're watching TV? Do this exercise during commercials and you can have a major decline in your waistline. This exercise involves simply holding in your tummy and tightening the ab muscles.

Muscles affected: Abdominal muscles in general, but mostly lower abs.

Sets and reps: Do this for as long as you can during a 30-second commercial, relax for the next commercial, tighten as long as you can during the next commercial spot and so on. You'll end up doing at least three or four tighten-up sessions during every commercial break, and many more if you're watching TBS Superstation. In fact, if you're watching TBS you may lose an inch off your waistline the first evening.

Checkpoints: Sit up straight while you are doing this, and breathe while you're tightening. The results you get from this exercise are in relation to the effort you put in, so suck and tighten!

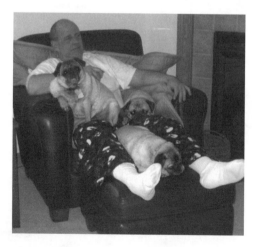

I'll mow the grass later...right now we're working on our abs!

Additional copies of this book can be ordered from
www.MADSfitness.com
www.FirstAmericanPublishing.com
or your favorite bookstore or online book seller